Boundaries of Care

Anthropology of Well-Being

Individual, Community, Society

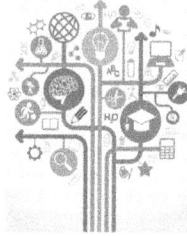

Series Editor: Ben G. Blount, PhD (SocioEcological Informatics)

Mission Statement

Well-being is central and important in people's daily lives and life history. This book series brings about understanding of what the complex concepts of well-being include. The concepts of quality of life, life satisfaction, and happiness will be explored and viewed at the individual level, the community level, and the level of society. The series encourages and promotes research into the concept of well-being, how it appears to be defined culturally, and how it is utilized across levels and across different social, economic, and ethnic groups. Understandings of how well-being promotes stability and resilience will also be critical to advances in understanding, as well as how well-being can be implemented as a goal in resisting vulnerabilities and in adaptation. Series books include monographs and edited collections by a range of academics, from rising scholars to experts in relevant fields.

Advisory Board Members

Steven Jacob, Kathleen Galvin, Carlos Garcia-Quijano, Cynthia Isenhour, and
Richard Pollnac

Recent Titles in the Series

Boundaries of Care: Community Health Workers in the United States, by Ryan I. Logan
Living with HIV in Post-Crisis Times: Beyond the Endgame, edited by David A.B. Murray
Diversity and Cultural Competence in the Health Sector: Ebola-Affected Countries in West Africa, by Mohamed Kanu, Elizabeth A. Williams, Charles Williams, and Regina Bash-Taqi
Everyday Food Practices: Commercialisation and Consumption in the Periphery of the Global North, by Tarunna Sebastian
No Perfect Birth: Trauma and Obstetric Care in the Rural United States, by Kristin Haltinner
Love and its Entanglements among the Enxet of Paraguay: Social and Kinship Relations within a Market Economy, by Stephen Kidd

Boundaries of Care

Community Health Workers in the United States

Ryan I. Logan

LEXINGTON BOOKS

Lanham • Boulder • New York • London

Published by Lexington Books
An imprint of The Rowman & Littlefield Publishing Group, Inc.
4501 Forbes Boulevard, Suite 200, Lanham, Maryland 20706
www.rowman.com

86-90 Paul Street, London EC2A 4NE

British Library Cataloguing in Publication Information Available

Library of Congress Cataloging-in-Publication Data

Names: Logan, Ryan I., author.
Title: Boundaries of care : community health workers in the United States / Ryan I. Logan.
Description: Lanham : Lexington Books, [2022] | Series: Anthropology of well-being: Individual, community, society | Includes bibliographical references and index.
Identifiers: LCCN 2021051300 (print) | LCCN 2021051301 (ebook) | ISBN 9781793629463 (cloth) | ISBN 9781793629487 (paperback) | ISBN 9781793629470 (ebook)
Subjects: LCSH: Community health services—United States. | Health promotion—United States.
Classification: LCC RA445 .L64 2022 (print) | LCC RA445 (ebook) | DDC 362.10973—dc23/eng/20211124
LC record available at https://lccn.loc.gov/2021051300
LC ebook record available at https://lccn.loc.gov/2021051301

Contents

List of Figures and Tables   vii

Preface   ix

Acknowledgments   xiii

Introduction: "Reaching Them Where They're At"   1

1 "There Is Hope Out There": Community Health Workers
and the Moral Economy of Care   23

2 Connecting with Clients and Engendering Empowerment:
Analyzing the CHW-Client Relationship   47

3 Present Yet Invisible: Issues of Exclusion and Inclusion in the
Professional Workforce   71

4 Boundaries of Care: How Caregiving Is Shaped in
Community Health Work   95

5 "So That No One Can Belittle Them": Advocacy
as Caregiving   117

6 "You Cannot Pour from an Empty Cup": Burnout,
Compassion Fatigue, and Self-Care   141

Conclusion   163

References   185

Index   203

About the Author   207

List of Figures and Tables

FIGURES

Figure 0.1 Map of Indiana   13

Figure 1.1 "Each of these doors, stairs, and halls have afforded
            me an opportunity . . . to meet a neighbor in need, in
            need of something, something that is always different,
            different but enlightening. Regardless of who is behind
            that door, up those stairs, or down the hall, these doors,
            stairs, and halls are thresholds to new relationships,
            steps to stronger communities and paths to healthier
            neighbors. Being a community health worker is not
            a duty, it is an opportunity to open closed doors, lift
            people to new heights, and brighten dimly lit halls—
            just like these doors, stairs, and halls have afforded me
            an opportunity"   34

Figure 1.2 "Many times you may be apprehensive about what you
            see and doubt whether or not you have the ability to
            help put the puzzle pieces together"   38

Figure 2.1 "A clearer picture can be seen when the blindfolds
            have been removed"   54

Figure 2.2 "One of our challenges is being valued by our clients
            because sometimes we provide our services for free"   67

Figure 3.1 "Overcoming the idea that the Land of Opportunity is
            for everyone"   85

Figure 4.1 "Must have big ears, big eyes, and a very,
            very small mouth"   100

Figure 5.1 "For me, being a CHW means advocating for others
            no matter their skin color, religion, economic status,
            or nationality"   119
Figure 5.2 Levels of CHW Advocacy and Specific Area of Impact   120
Figure 5.3 "Helping patients know how to jump into the health
            care system"   124

TABLES

Table 0.1 Community Health Worker Competencies and Examples   8
Table 0.2 Demographic Characteristics of the CHW Sample   15
Table 3.1 Adapted List of Terms for CHWs from the Indiana
           State Department of Health   76
Table 5.1 Examples of CHW Advocacy at Each Level   121

Preface

While Indiana may not come to the minds of many as a location for an anthropological field site, my deep connection to the state served as an anchor to develop the ethnographic research project described in this book. My family moved to Indiana in 1994 when I was a young child and I spent the majority of my formative years there. While completing my undergraduate degree in Anthropology and, later, a master's degree in Applied Anthropology at Indiana University-Purdue University Indianapolis (IUPUI), I read many ethnographies and academic articles written by anthropologists in far off, "exotic" places. However, I had been instilled by my tremendous anthropology professors at IUPUI to turn the anthropological gaze inward, at our own state, environment and society. In my training as an undergraduate and graduate student at IUPUI, I participated in many projects that were based within Indianapolis and in various regions of Indiana.

Given my connection to this state, in late 2015, I began thinking of a compelling research project I could conduct within Indiana—a project that would be focused on health, health disparities, marginalized populations, and a unique group of healthcare providers called community health workers (CHWs). In choosing Indiana as a field site, I argue—in the same vein as my professors, and, now, as I tell my own students—that we should always be turning our anthropological gaze inward—at our society and at ourselves—and start from the ground up as we explore pertinent cultural and social issues that the discipline of anthropology can illuminate. In the paragraphs that follow, I provide some insight to the reader into the beginning of the project described in this book, how the project impacted me as a researcher, and how the participants have left their mark in this book.

Although I was bundled up, I was still shivering in 20-degree Fahrenheit weather in the morning of February 27, 2017, in northwest Indiana—barely a 30-minute drive from Chicago—as I waited at the front of a hotel with several other CHWs. We were headed to the first day of an intensive, weeklong CHW certification course. I was a bit apprehensive and unsure what to expect. The community partner organization, with whom I was collaborating with, had made an exception in allowing me to undergo the new CHW certification course (given my interest in conducting a collaborative research project on the topic of CHWs) with several other CHWs who would later become key informants in the research. While this will be further explained throughout the book, the certification was being implemented as one key step to incorporate CHWs into the professional workforce. Being part of this certification course provided me with unique insight into the new certification course in addition to learning the finer points and nuances of the training CHWs would begin receiving following the official rollout of this course later in 2017. What I learned in the certification course left an indelible impact on myself—not only in terms of my experience as a researcher but also as a professor.

Throughout this project, I was embedded in the CHW movement in Indiana, which also resulted in transformative changes to myself. Little did I know at the moment that this training would change how I teach and interact with my future students. My training as a CHW shifted my way of thinking—in terms of utilizing informal counseling and motivational interviewing with advisees, locating and connecting students to resources, serving as a source of support, and advocating for students. My experience during this project transformed me from an interested party in the success of my students to an active party that seeks the best for them. Thus, this research project contributed to positive changes that have shaped me for the better. The subsequent sections of this book will elaborate on how CHWs learn and employ these same techniques in their quest to improve the health and well-being of their clients and communities.

Additionally, this monograph was the result of years of thought, collaboration, and research with CHWs in Indiana spanning from the beginning in 2016 with pilot research, the main data collection period between June 2017 through April 2018, follow-up research in the summer of 2019, and ongoing data collection via Zoom throughout 2020 and 2021. As an applied, critical medical anthropologist, I sought to collaborate with participants, produce applicable research findings, and contribute to theoretical debates in the discipline of anthropology. It is my hope that the findings presented in this book produce far-reaching impacts. The ethnographic text in the book provides rich insights into the lived experiences of CHWs in Indiana, theoretical contributions, and practical steps that can be taken by policy-makers and other stakeholders to better understand these workers and to implement in policy change to enhance, recognize, and support this workforce. The book itself contributes to the disciplines of medical anthropology and public health in addition to demonstrating useful concepts that can be applied in CHW movements throughout the United States and the world.

Finally, elevating the voices of participants has been an integral part of this ongoing project. The community partners and partner organization took an active role in the design, data collection, and analysis phases of this project. Through the method of photovoice, participants produced and interpreted findings that further illustrated the lived experiences of these workers. Several participants took part in a focus group interview to assess the initial data analysis and offered their critiques and feedback. Three other key informants continued their participation in graciously giving their time to reviewing the original version of this manuscript and offered additional feedback, critiques, and corrections. This book would not have come to fruition without the collaboration between myself and the community partners.

All proceeds from this book will be donated to the CHW movement in Indiana.

Acknowledgments

This book is first and foremost dedicated to the community health workers and the research participants who made this project possible. Your tireless efforts to help your clients and communities improve their health are admirable and the possibilities you bring to their lives are limitless. Thank you all for taking me under your wing and showing me your world. Many of you took an active role during data collection and offered critiques and further insights into the data analysis and earlier drafts of this book all of which have enriched this final product. Though I cannot thank you all by name due to confidentiality, without you this book would not have been possible. Thank you.

This book would also not have been possible without the years of support and mentorship from a variety of individuals. Dr. Heide Castañeda, thank you for all of your time, support, and mentorship. You've left an indelible impact on my life, career, and outlook. I'm eternally thankful for the time you took reviewing and offering feedback on earlier drafts of this manuscript. I also want to thank Drs. Tara Deubel, Lisa Staten, Nancy Romero-Daza, and Kevin Yelvington for your help and support over the years. Drs. Wendy Vogt and Susan Hyatt, thank you so much for your continued support and mentorship throughout my time as an undergraduate student, graduate student, and into my professional career. Many others at Indiana University-Purdue University Indianapolis (IUPUI) were key sources of inspiration and support over the years including Drs. Paul Mullins, Jeanette Dickerson-Putman, Larry Zimmerman, Gina Sánchez-Gibau, and Jeremy Wilson. I will always owe a debt of gratitude to Dr. Kelly M. Branam who first introduced me to anthropology back in my freshman semester at IUPUI in 2007. I'm also thankful for the friendship, encouragement, and support of my colleagues at California State University, Stanislaus—especially Drs. S. Steve Arounsack, Richard

H. Wallace, Ellen E. Bell, Sari Miller-Antonio, Jeffrey Frost, José R. Díaz-Garayúa, Thomas Durbin, and many others. I also owe a big thanks to Robert Shepherd for reviewing, editing, and offering feedback on this manuscript. Lastly, I want to offer a sincerest thank you to Jerry Brickley. It was in your high school English classes that I first discovered my love of research and writing, thank you Mr. Brickley!

I am also grateful to my academic colleagues and friends. I want to especially thank Kanan Mehta, Laura Kihlström, Seiichi Villalona, and Olubukola Olayiwola for supporting and helping me grow over the years. I'm also indebted to Linda Clark for the support and friendship. To my other colleagues and friends at the University of South Florida, thank you for all of your help and support over the years. In no particular order, I'd like to thank Ted Gold, Carla Castillo, Dana Ketcher, Laura Leisinger, Hadi Khoshneviss, Sarita Panchang, Kevin Smiley, Mika Kadono, Aria Walsh-Felz, Lia Berman, Jacqueline Sivén, Sami Sivén, Melissa Sedlacik, and Atte Penttilä,

I'm very grateful to Kasey Beduhn of Lexington Books at Rowman and Littlefield Publishing Group. Thank you for initially reaching out and contacting me at the American Anthropological Association Annual Conference in Vancouver in 2019 to inquire about the research I was presenting—that initial email led to this book. I am also indebted to the anonymous reviewer for their feedback and thoughts on the manuscript, which helped me further strengthen and refine the arguments and findings presented in this book. I am also thankful to the production team at Lexington Books at Rowman and Littlefield Publishing Group. Various arguments from chapters 3 and 5 have appeared in Logan, Ryan I. "Professionalization as a 'Double-Edged Sword': Assessing the Professional Citizenship of Community Health Workers in the Midwest." *Human Organization* 80, no. 3 (2021): 192–202, and Logan, Ryan I. "Being A Community Health Worker Means Advocating: Participation, Perceptions, and Challenges in Advocacy." *Anthropology in Action* 26, no. 2 (2019): 9–18, respectively.

Finally, this book would not have been possible without the support of my friends and family. To my mother, Cathy S. Logan, thank you for your unconditional love and support. I miss you every day. To my father, Damian J. Logan, thank you for your steadfast support over all of these years. To my sister, Renny K. Monday, thank you for always being there and supporting me. To my wife, Paola A. Gonzalez, thank you for your tireless support, dedication, and always pushing me to be a better person. This book certainly would not have been finished without your encouragement and support. I want to thank the Gonzalez family, including Juan Carlos, Maria, Juan Camilo, and Carlos Felipe. I'm also thankful to Christopher D. Monday and Andrés Guevara for their support and friendship over the years. I also owe a special thanks to Patti and Dan Anderson for their tremendous support and encouragement. Finally, I owe thanks to many friends who have given me countless support, laughter, and friendship over the years including Michael Lingeman, Daniel Roman, Steven Roman, Brian Spony, Joe English, Troy Blackport, Jeff Cann, and Nathan Francis. To the countless others who I have not named, thank you!

Introduction

"Reaching Them Where They're At"

It was early morning and already a hot and humid Indiana summer. I was driving to northwest Indiana—colloquially known as "The Region," a nick-name stemming from the Calumet (River) Region. This area sits along the Illinois and Michigan borders and comprises cities such as Gary, Hammond, and East Chicago, home to large minority populations including African Americans and Latinx immigrants who experience social inequality, racism, and structural violence[1] as exhibited by lead in the drinking water,[2] lack of jobs,[3] and reduced access to health resources. As this book will show, The Region is one such area that could significantly benefit further incorporation of community health workers (CHWs), defined by the CHW Section of the American Public Health Association[4] as a

> frontline public health worker who is a trusted member of and/or has an unusu-ally close understanding of the community served. This trusting relationship enables the worker to serve as a liaison/link/intermediary between health/social services and the community to facilitate access to services and improve the qual-ity and cultural competence of service delivery.

I was traveling to meet with two CHWs: Martha[5]—an indefatigable Black woman and educator in her 70s—and Leticia—a middle-aged Latinx woman who had previously worked as a registered nurse. Together, they had more than two decades of experience as CHWs, and they were also key figures in the rollout and design of a newly minted CHW certification course. I met them several months prior during my time as a student in the course. Both work for a faith-based, non-profit public health organization. Martha, Leticia, and other members of the organization conduct regular outreach to the community, advocate for their clients, develop partnerships with other

1

community-based organizations, and work to counter health disparities. Their organization is located off a major highway and surrounded by warehouses, auto shops, and other repair shops; nonetheless, it is a prime location for quickly getting around The Region to connect with the local community.

Martha and I talked about the challenges facing CHWs, especially their lack of official recognition and broad acceptance as distinct members of the professional workforce. Martha identified a crucial issue both in Indiana and throughout the United States, stating that "for Indiana especially, the shortage of healthcare workers is beginning to be a challenge because we have doctors and nurses that are retiring." She continued,

> [There's] gotta be an entry into it [the workforce]. CHWs could be that health educator or member of a healthcare team that follows a patient . . . that helps them from relapsing or being admitted to a hospital because they didn't know how to manage their chronic condition.

Martha emphasized that health education and helping clients[6] *outside* of the hospital is where CHWs especially contribute to care. "That's where I see a great importance for CHWs, to be that educator where the doctor or nurse doesn't have the time to do that. . . . They [medical professionals] cannot hand-hold, but the CHW could possibly help that individual." It is precisely at this juncture where CHWs improve health—through education, advocacy, and connection of clients to resources. Martha summarized, "The CHW could focus on the individual client and help them not go back into the system."

Just one month prior to my meeting with Martha and Leticia, I had met with Carmen, a Black woman fluent in Spanish and Portuguese. Carmen was unique as a CHW in that she had an advanced degree and had formerly worked as a scientist. She quickly became a key interlocuter throughout the duration of the project detailed in this book. Though technically employed as a *promotora* (literally, "health promoter," a Spanish-speaking CHW), she also works as a medical interpreter. During our first of many discussions, Carmen related to me how she spends her free time volunteering within her community in South Central Indiana, helping clients fill out paperwork for benefits, advocating on their behalf, and helping meet or finding ways to meet their needs. One situation that she had recently experienced had particularly upset her. Carmen described how she had found one of her clients—a 71-year-old Vietnam veteran with type 2 diabetes—to be uninsured and uncertain about how he would get the insulin he desperately needed. When she asked him if he had insulin, the veteran told her, "I know how to make it stretch." Frustrated that her elderly client was not on Medicare[7]—he had, it seemed, fallen through the cracks of the U.S. healthcare system—Carmen exclaimed, "How was a caseworker missing this guy? That's what I'm saying—reaching them where they're at." Carmen continued, "And then I see people say 'How we love our veterans!' That's the stuff that drives me bats." While upsetting, her story was one of many similar ones that I encountered in my interactions with CHWs. Carmen's story, and the many detailed in this book, underscore the need for these workers within the U.S. healthcare system.

Research with CHWs has produced an extensive body of literature related to the positive health outcomes resulting from their activities, the potential for their work to increase the cost-effectiveness of health care, and other benefits of integration of CHWs into the healthcare and social services work-forces.[8] However, few studies—if any—have taken a long-term, ethnographic approach to document the lived experience of these workers in the United States. Overall, this book contributes to furthering our understanding of the realities and complexities of CHWs in the United States through examining the nuances of their lived experiences and the myriad forces that shape their caregiving.

PRESENT YET INVISIBLE

Even before the COVID-19 pandemic, the U.S. healthcare system faced two dire issues: too few healthcare workers[9] and burgeoning health disparities.[10] CHWs address gaps in care that exist due to racism and unequal access through direct outreach to clients and providing care outside of the clinic—thus encapsulating Carmen's notion of "reaching them where they are at." A primary rationale of the project detailed in this book was to highlight how CHWs are *present yet invisible* in the healthcare workforce in the United States, and in Indiana, in particular. Despite the fact that CHWs have a history going back more than half a century, in many parts of the United States, medical professionals and the public seem unaware of their presence. Indiana is one such state where a lack of awareness of CHWs is common. However, as I will demonstrate, their roles are requisite and thus this book introduces readers to their caregiving and opportunities for greater inclusion of CHWs in the healthcare system in the United States and globally.

At the time of my research for this book, a statewide CHW organization, the Community Health Workers' Organization of Indiana[11] (CHWOI), began rolling out a certification in addition to helping develop policy related to CHWs through extensive collaboration with the state government. This culminated in their official recognition, yet other ramifications emerged regarding their professionalization, as this book will discuss. I divided my time across as much of the state as possible, visiting with CHWs in northeast, southeast, southern, southwest, and central Indiana. During interviews and while shadowing these workers, I witnessed how CHWs care for their clients and communities. The findings—as interpreted by myself and the CHW participants—revealed the complex and intricate ways in which CHWs connect with clients, engage with their broader communities, and provide care. This book explains why CHWs are seemingly present yet invisible and, in illuminating their lived experiences, highlights the nuances of their caregiving, demonstrates their dedication, details the challenges that arise via professionalization, and illustrates the significant contributions they make to the overall healthcare landscape.

THE BOUNDARIES OF (AND BARRIERS TO) CARE

A prominent theme of this book are the *boundaries of and barriers* CHWs faced in their caregiving. The boundaries manifested in a variety of physical locations, including the environment, doctor's offices, and social service agencies. Other times, boundaries coalesced in the form of intangible abstractions including laws, policies, scope of care, structural violence, exclusion from the professional workforce, and conceptions of deservingness. Regardless of how they manifest, these boundaries presented a challenge for CHWs to either (1) remain within the designated guidelines and acquiesce to the boundary or (2) choose to cross said boundary in pursuit of care for their client(s) and communities. In confronting these boundaries, CHWs drew on their knowledge of resources, training, skills, competencies, and participation in advocacy—the latter of which serves in and of itself as a form of caregiving.

At times, however, CHWs encountered barriers that prevented them from providing services, procuring needed resources, or navigating the professional landscape within which they worked. Other barriers manifested within the CHW-client relationship, within the medical community, and within the broader public. These resulted in complications in the provision of care and hindered or impaired the connection between CHWs and their clients. This relationship is particularly delicate and built on profound trust—from which the CHW and client worked together to improve well-being. Other barriers occurred from a lack of professional integration that complicated the ability of CHWs to provide care to their fullest ability. This book reveals how, in their caregiving, these workers navigated, crossed, or were hindered by these boundaries and barriers.

The boundaries and barriers described throughout this book highlight the complex nuances of the work and caregiving provided by CHWs in addition to the resiliency, ingenuity, and dedication of these workers. They are pressured in competing directions: staying within boundaries could be laudatory for following guidelines, laws, and procedures, or push against and cross boundaries and barriers, often via advocacy or activism, and by doing so improve the health and well-being of their clients and communities. In both ways, boundaries and barriers framed the daily lives of these workers and their caregiving.

A BRIEF OVERVIEW OF CHWS

CHWs are members of the health and social services workforce and have typically, in the United States, operated on the margins of the established healthcare teams (e.g., comprised of doctors, physician assistants, registered nurses, medical assistants, and social workers). In addition to this definition, the APHA[12] further defines a CHW as someone who "builds individual and community capacity by increasing health knowledge and self-sufficiency through a range of activities such as outreach, community education, informal counseling, social support and advocacy." This definition highlights the unique skill set that CHWs possess, one that sets them apart from other established members of the healthcare team, particularly given their outreach work that occurs outside the walls of clinics.

These workers typically excel at understanding and addressing the social determinants of health that manifest as disparities for marginalized populations. These social determinants include, but are not limited to, a lack of transportation, financial capital, health insurance, food security, and physical safety. These disparities complicate the ability of individuals to achieve health and well-being and exercise an increased burden within marginalized populations including Black, Latinx, Asian, Indigenous, immigrant, refugee, and individuals experiencing homelessness, mental health disorders, and/or substance use disorders.

Through their participation in advocacy, outreach, health education, motivational interviewing, and informal counseling, CHWs are well-suited to address the myriad issues that complicate care outside of the hospital and clinic. Their genesis extends back at least a century, with many scholars identifying their origin in the 1920s with the formalization of the "barefoot doctors" of China.[13] Barefoot doctors were peasants trained in basic medical skills and tasked with providing care to China's significant rural population, expected to spend half of their time providing basic medical care and the other half working in agriculture.[14] In the 1960s, the barefoot doctor model proliferated to other countries to address the healthcare needs of impoverished populations throughout the world, particularly in Asia, Africa, and Latin America (with workers in the latter region being known as *promotores* [*de salud*], literally, "health promoters"). The *promotor* model combined Catholic liberation theology—a religious and social movement that aimed to empower the poor against their oppressors—and labor rights struggles.[15]

CHWs found their official footing in the United States in the 1960s as part of the Great Society programs championed by President Lyndon B. Johnson.[16] CHW programs received federal funds in the Federal Migrant Health Act of 1962 and the Economic Opportunity Act of 1964.[17] Several years later, in 1968, the Indian Health Service founded a CHW program to provide services in Indigenous communities in the United States.[18] Although the following decades would see a disinterest in CHW programs, this was reversed in the 1990s as their value within migrant farmworker communities became evident. During these decades, CHWs promoted social justice for marginalized communities.[19] CHWs, as their counterparts in Latin America, sought to not only improve health but to address social injustices, which are intimately connected to well-being.

While support for CHW programs has waxed and waned since their inception, CHWs have been ever-present. Some states, such as Arizona, Minnesota, and Oregon, have successfully integrated CHWs into their workforce and have even provided institutional support such as Medicaid reimbursement for CHW services.[20] However, in many parts of the United States, these workers remain on the periphery of the health and social services workforce. Nationally, the U.S. Bureau of Labor Statistics[21] estimates that there are 56,130 CHWs employed in the United States. Other estimates put the range of individuals functioning as CHWs within the United States between 85,000 and 200,000.[22] Globally, conservative estimates place the number of CHWs at 5 million, with as many as 2.3 million operating in India alone.[23]

CHWs throughout the globe face similar issues, including ones related to safety, pay, and complications resulting from their professionalization.[24] In various countries, a lack of policies that support CHWs has led to issues related to remuneration, lack of care coordination, protests for increased labor protections, and moonlighting.[25] Research has documented how professionalization has resulted in the formation of CHW hierarchies that have in turn resulted in tensions within the workforce,[26] while other work has analyzed how neighborly relations and belongingness within their communities inform and affect the care provided by CHWs.[27]

Despite these issues, numerous studies have demonstrated the efficacy of CHWs, including their positive impacts on the management of chronic disease, diminishment of the impact of health disparities in marginalized populations, provision of essential input to health research, and improvement of overall access to health care both globally and throughout the United States.[28] In addition, these workers can produce cost-effective outcomes.[29] In spite of these benefits, the professional status of these workers varies greatly from country to country, regionally, and throughout the United States.

THE CONTEXT OF CARE: CHWS IN INDIANA

CHWs have an extensive history in Indiana going back at least 30 years. Many of these workers have provided their services under a variety of different titles, which has complicated and delayed their recognition within the professional workforce and broader public. In 2011, the Indiana State Department of Health began a project to understand and define CHWs, followed by a series of statewide meetings that sought to develop this workforce. In the following year, a CHW coalition was formed that conducted surveys in both English and Spanish to understand these workers better throughout the state. The coalition launched social media sites and held a meeting to share the findings of the survey results, which served to define and organize the CHW movement in Indiana.

Law passed at the federal level engendered discussions of the role of CHWs in Indiana. The Patient Protection and Affordable Care Act (ACA) passed in 2010 marked a shift in the healthcare landscape of the United States. Though not perfect, it expanded healthcare access to millions; referenced CHWs by name; and highlighted the potential contributions of CHWs to the healthcare workforce, the potential for Medicaid reimbursement for CHW services, and potential sources of funding.[30] Although these funding streams failed to materialize, the recognition of these workers brought renewed interest in their potential. Later, in 2015, Indiana became one of the few politically conservative states to expand Medicaid via the ACA. The Medicaid expansion[31] was significant as it provided health insurance to many who had been previously uninsured.[32]

A couple of years prior to the Medicaid expansion, in 2013, the CHW coalition emerged as the CHWOI. The organization appointed a board of directors and a president in addition to dividing the state into ten regions based on health needs, demographics, and geography. The goals of this organization are to unite CHWs throughout Indiana, to amplify the voices of these workers, and to advocate for their recognition and advancement. CHWOI organizes CHWs throughout the state and collaborates with universities and public health organizations to conduct research, provide training opportunities to CHWs, deliver health and social service resources to those in need, and collaborate with local, state, and federal politicians.

Over the next several years, CHWOI developed a strategic plan, appointed regional directors to oversee issues in the ten demarcated regions of Indiana, and began developing a plan to become the certifying body of CHWs in the state. The organization continued building its network of CHWs, reviewing certification programs and refining its own certification program for Indiana. In 2017, the certification course was given to a small group of CHWs to test and review the final curriculum. These individuals would then serve as master trainers, through CHWOI, to teach the curriculum to CHWs throughout the state.

The certification course was largely adapted from a curriculum of another large, Midwestern public health organization. The course is meant to provide a foundational education in skills, competencies, roles, and scope of care for CHWs (see table 0.1 for specific details on CHW competencies). The course is 70 hours in total and the cost for enrollment is currently $1,500. The classes are a combination of lecture, video clips, discussion, textbook reading, activities that provide students with academic and practical issues, and opportunities to role-play in a safe environment to practice and hone their skills. The course is taught by two CHW instructors who have been certified by and are affiliated with CHWOI. The classes are also adaptable to the needs of the students, with the course sometimes being offered over two, nonconsecutive weeks (in approximately daily 8-hour classes) or over the course of a month (in approximately daily 4-hour classes). Following the onset of the COVID-19 pandemic, the course was adapted, in 2020, to be taught virtually in a

Table 0.1   Community Health Worker Competencies and Examples

Competency	Examples
Communication Skills	Ability to communicate clearly, culturally appropriate language, listening skills
Interpersonal and Relationship-Building Skills	Manage conflict, motivational interviewing, self-management coaching
Service Coordination and Navigation Skills	Make appropriate referrals, coordinate CHW activities, follow-up with clients
Capacity-Building Skills	Help clients identify goals, work toward community empowerment, community organizing
Advocacy Skills	Advocate for policies to improve community health, identify barriers to care, promote change
Education and Facilitation Skills	Utilize culturally appropriate educational strategies to improve health and well-being
Individual and Community Assessment Skills	Participate in individual and community assessments
Outreach Skills	Identify resources, connect with those in need, build a resources inventory
Professional Skills and Conduct	Set goals and develop a work plan, manage time, set boundaries, and practice self-care
Evaluation and Research Skills	Assist, support, and contribute to evaluation and research
Knowledge Base	Be knowledgeable about social determinants of health, public health principles, community served

synchronous format (that occurs live, utilizing videoconferencing and chat) via the Zoom application.

Shortly after the rollout of the CHW certification course, the governor of Indiana, Eric Holcomb, convened a CHW task force that held its first meeting in October 2017. The goals of this group were to define the roles, responsibilities, and competencies of CHWs in Indiana; determine the certification process for these workers; and decide on a set of CHW-specific, Medicaid reimbursable services. The primary thrust would be to provide CHWs, finally, with an avenue into the medical and social services workforce via this process of professionalization—encapsulated by the certification and by CHW-specific services being Medicaid reimbursable.

The task force was made up of 15 members from a variety of stakeholder groups, including representatives from the Indiana State Department of Health, the Department of Workforce Development, the Office of Medicaid Policy and Planning, mental health organizations, and other statewide health organizations. This task force included *one* CHW— the president of CHWOI, Lucía – who was vital in providing experience, background, and knowledge. This lack of CHW representation and thus opportunity for CHWs to maintain control over the very process of the official characterization of their field is indicative of the ongoing problem in their recognition and status among politicians, bureaucrats, and healthcare professionals, generally. Lucía's participation in this task force was essential in that she provided other task force members with clear understandings of what a CHW is and of the core roles and functions of these workers. Additionally, she drew on extensive research conducted with CHWs throughout the state and through her collaborations to amplify their voices in these meetings. Though technically the task force still exists, in December 2018 it stopped meeting once there was agreement on the agenda items it had set for itself. While the professionalization of these workers removed some boundaries, they still encountered a variety of challenges as later chapters will show.

This book provides a simultaneous top-down and bottom-up examination of the lives of CHWs in Indiana. The findings presented herein are timely, given that nationwide, these workers are (and have) gaining(ed) distinct membership as part of established healthcare teams consisting of medical doctors, physician assistants, nurses, therapists, and social workers. Furthermore, one objective of this book is to hasten this process by illustrating how the work of CHWs complements that of other medical paraprofessionals, including doulas, case managers, and home healthcare workers. Overall, these workers fill a niche by promoting health outside the doctor's office via their community outreach, health education, informal counseling, and advocacy.

FRAMING THE LIVED EXPERIENCES
OF CHWS IN INDIANA

This book elucidates the wide range of lived experiences encountered by CHWs, from their motivations, relationships developed with clients and the broader community, their experiences with burnout, and the (health) impacts of their advocacy. I draw upon several key theoretical lenses that frame the nuances and complexities regarding the professional and lived experiences of CHWs. Thereby, this book highlights rich, ethnographic details that contribute not only to an academic understanding of these workers but also applied insights that can be utilized by employers, public health programs, and CHW organizations to better understand and operationalize this workforce.

Undeniably, the relationships CHWs fostered with their clients and community were key for participants in this study and their raison d'être. The ethnographic findings presented reveal how CHWs structure their identity, their relationships with clients, and how this motivates them to provide aid to their clients (see chapters 1 and 2). Moral economy serves as a lens for examining, understanding, and analyzing how CHWs function within their communities. This framework analyzes how morals, obligations, motivations, and ethics shape and determine relationships, interactions, and exchanges between and among individuals. The origination of this theory is credited to historian E. P. Thompson[33] and anthropologist James Scott.[34] Thompson defined moral economy as "social norms and obligations, of the proper economic functions of several parties within the community."[35] Moral economy has since gone through several iterations and has been utilized in a variety of anthropological studies as well as informing research with CHWs.[36]

In particular, I draw on Didier Fassin's reinterpretation of this framework, which he defines as "the production, distribution, circulation, and utilization of moral sentiments, emotions, and values, norms, and obligation in the social space."[37] Since CHWs typically come from the communities they serve, moral economy serves as a lens to reveal the nuances and forces that shape their lived experiences. These workers are motivated by their morals, values, and obligations to their communities and clients and thus participate in a moral economy of care. As such, this theoretical lens reveals insights into micro-level forces that shape relationships in addition to assessing the impacts of the broader political economic context. CHWs leverage their commitment and relationships built with clients to provide resources and empower clients to take charge of their health and well-being. However, an important critique must be levied because, through such relationships, CHWs can inadvertently reproduce the neoliberal economic approach in their caregiving—which is pervasive in the U.S. healthcare system. This approach emphasizes that the individual is solely responsible for their health and health choices. While individual health behaviors are but one component which shapes health, environmental factors—in the form of social determinants of health (e.g., employment status, income, access to health care, food insecurity, language, discrimination, etc.)—are crucial to consider. However, as detailed in chapter 2, CHWs mitigate a neoliberal approach to health while also circumventing and actively working to ameliorate the negative effects of the social determinants of health.

CHWs and their communities experience varying levels of structural vulnerability. This theoretical model was proposed by Quesada et al., who describe this vulnerability as a positionality that "is produced by his or her location in a hierarchical social order and its diverse networks of power relationships and affects."[38] CHWs experience structural vulnerability based on their race, ethnicity, sex, and, for immigrant CHWs, legal status. Additionally, the majority of CHWs are women (up to 70 percent worldwide,[39] 82 percent in the United States,[40] and 80 percent of participants in this study) and many are women of color (67 percent of participants in this study). As this book will show, structural vulnerability impacts this workforce, which negatively affects their ability to navigate the professional workforce, procure resources for their communities, and provide care to clients.

Medical citizenship also provides the necessary framing for understanding how the state structures access to care for CHWs and their communities. This theory is defined as "how membership in a state, a society, or even humanity itself is mediated by prevailing regimes of health-related power and knowledge."[41] This framework elucidates how individuals and groups are denied or afforded equal access to health care and resources—and, thus, who is accorded citizenship, considered as belonging or unbelonging, and deserving (or, undeserving). This lens reveals the constellation of factors that create and perpetuate health disparities and injustices in the communities served by these workers. CHWs, in the majority of cases, come from the communities they serve (or may be individuals in recovery and/or have their own mental health disorders) and have experienced structural violence and marginalization in their personal lives. This violence also becomes reproduced in their professional lives.

Analyzing and understanding the impacts regarding the professionalization of CHWs in Indiana served as a primary component of this project. Although Lucía's membership was vital, the task force remained woefully lacking in terms of CHW representation throughout its existence. This lack of representation in the task force, in addition to condescension, various challenges, and heavy workloads exemplifies both the structural vulnerability and the lack of citizenship experienced by CHWs. Building on medical citizenship, I introduce the concept of *professional citizenship*, defined as "the belongingness and legitimacy of a group within the workforce."[42] This analytical lens reveals issues of belonging and legitimacy, as well as ramifications that arise via the process of professionalization. This lens is supported by "legitimizing mechanisms," which facilitate belongingness, recognition, and/or foster legitimacy. These mechanisms can include earning a professional certification, increasing awareness of the position within the professional workforce and the general public, completing specialty trainings or earning additional certifications (e.g., midwifery, doula, lactation consultant, nutrition, chronic disease management), and performing Medicaid reimbursable services. Professional citizenship provides recognition, legitimacy, and acceptance for CHWs but also comes at a cost in terms of potential ramifications described in this book.

Ultimately, these framings provide clarity to the lived experiences of CHWs and their caregiving, successes, challenges, and resiliency. Despite their own structural vulnerability, participants in this sample emerged as leaders in their communities and worked to circumvent the social determinants of health and the political economic context of Indiana to improve health and overall well-being. As such, these framings and the resultant analyses presented in this book contribute to academic and applied understandings of these workers and underscores the requisite nature of CHWs.

THE FIELD SITE: INDIANA

The research detailed in this book was conducted throughout Indiana, with participants interviewed in both rural and urban settings. Indiana (see figure 0.1) is a large and increasingly diverse state with a population of 6.7 million.[43] Indiana's population is approximately 84 percent White, 10 percent Black, 7 percent Latinx, and 2 percent Asian.[44] The state is also home to a growing population of immigrants. The foreign-born population has consistently grown over the past three decades from 1.7 percent in 1990 to 3.1 percent in 2000 and to 4.9 percent in 2017.[45] Two of Indiana's largest cities, Indianapolis and Fort Wayne, have large populations of refugees from Myanmar.[46] The major countries of origin for Indiana's immigrant population include Mexico (31.6 percent), India (9.1 percent), China (7.9 percent), the Philippines (3.3 percent), and Myanmar (2.9 percent).[47] The Latinx population of Indiana has also grown over the past three decades from 1.8 percent in 1990 to 6.4 percent in 2014.[48] Additionally, in terms of undocumented immigration, there are an estimated 100,000 undocumented immigrants in Indiana.[49] Over a quarter of the population of Indianapolis—the capital and largest city in Indiana—is Black (28.6 percent in 2019).[50] These growing populations—often marginalized by and within the health and social services systems—can be significantly assisted by CHWs.

While there is an increasingly diverse population growing in the state, Indiana has not always been a welcoming environment—standing in stark

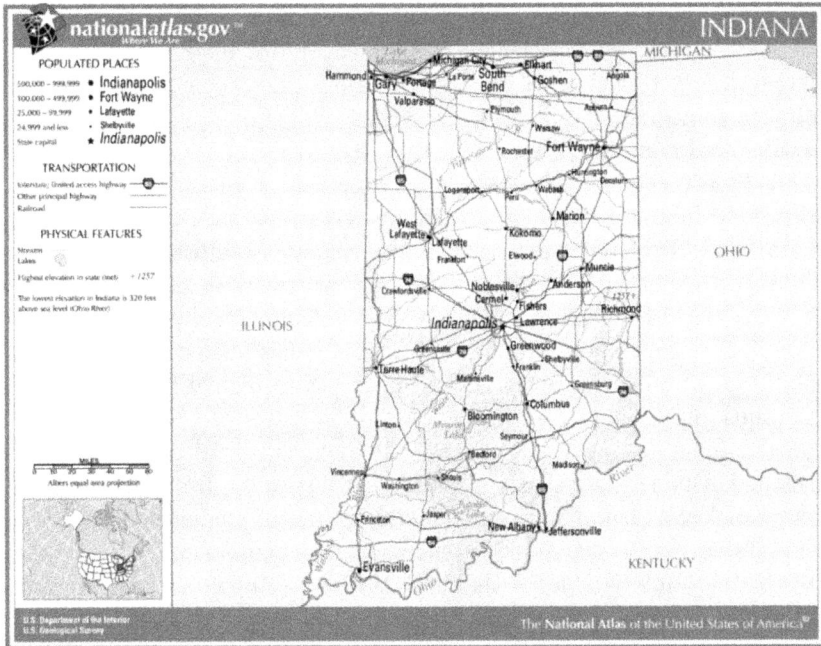

Figure 0.1   Map of Indiana. *Source: National Atlas of the United States.* Map of Indiana. 1970 Print Edition. Public domain.

contrast to its slogan of "Hoosier hospitality."[51] In August 2017, I drove to a major metropolitan area located in southwestern Indiana to meet with and shadow several CHWs. During my stay, I met with Mark, a well-dressed, middle-aged man who described himself as being "in recovery." A former probation officer turned CHW, Mark also served as an executive director of a community-based organization. He described how Indiana is both a "blessing and a curse" in regard to how it treats newcomers and marginalized populations, stating

> Indiana has good values and is about family and community but a lot of times we don't really appreciate multicultural or minority groups . . . immigrants, even the LGBT population. They usually have a pretty good fight on their hands in this state. So, I think on the one hand we're about family values but I think it's [Indiana] more 'traditional' so it's kind of a blessing and a curse.

Indiana has indeed been a hostile political environment for immigrant and LGBTQ+ populations. All 92 counties in the state participated in the Secure Communities program that targeted undocumented immigrants.[52] This program spans federal, state, and local law enforcement agencies that share information with Immigration and Customs Enforcement (ICE) in order to deport detained undocumented immigrants. While the program was discontinued in 2014 and replaced with the Priority Enforcement Program, the Trump administration reinstated the Secure Communities program via an executive order in 2017.

The LGBTQ+ population has also experienced structural violence in Indiana. In March 2015, legislation passed by then-governor Mike Pence would have allowed businesses and individuals to refuse service to the LGBTQ+ population. The law received national backlash and was amended to remove the discriminatory components in the subsequent weeks. However, the LGBTQ+ population of Indiana still faces issues related to employment, inability to afford medical care, lack of access to mental health care, and discrimination.[53]

In addition to its hostile political climate, Indiana consistently ranks as one of the unhealthiest states. Before the start of this study, from 2012 to 2015, Indiana ranked 41 out of 50 in terms of overall health.[54] Indiana raised its rank to 38 during pilot research and primary data collection from 2016 through 2018 but then fell back to its spot at 41. Additionally, other specific health indicators are poor—some worse than Indiana's overall rank. These health, social, and environmental issues include obesity (40), diabetes (41), smoking (41), public health funding[55] (48), preventable hospitalizations (40), mental health providers (43), primary care providers (34), infant mortality (43), frequent mental distress (35),[56] and frequent physical distress (36).[57]

Chronic disease, smoking, infant mortality, and drug use are significant health issues for Indiana. Specific disorders, diseases, and other health problems found in significant percentages of Indiana's population include diabetes (12.5 percent), obesity (34.1 percent), cardiovascular deaths (282.6 per 100,000), and smoking (21.1 percent).[58] The opioid crisis has also significantly impacted Indiana. Deaths associated with this crisis rose from 16.7 to 17.9 per 100,000 in 2017 to 20.2 per 100,000 in 2018 to 23.7 per 100,000 in 2019.[59] Minority populations (including Asian, Black, Indigenous, and Latinx communities) face health disparities related to sexually transmitted infections,[60] low birth weight,[61] premature death,[62] poor or fair health,[63] and children living in poverty.[64] Significantly, these specific health issues that often impact individuals outside the clinic or hospital walls can be ameliorated or at least diminished via risk reduction through interventions by CHWs.

THE STUDY

The findings presented in this book come from four years of ethnographic research in Indiana. In 2016, I established contact with Lucía, who was enthusiastic about conducting a research project on CHWs and we set out to incorporate the organization's research interests in conjunction with my own and vice versa. The collaborative aspect of this project was a crucial component of the research, helping me to collect data that could be used both to aid in policy development and to provide further insights into the CHW workforce in Indiana. Primary data collection for this project lasted from June 2017 to April 2018. Follow-up research was conducted sporadically from May 2019 through November 2021. I drew upon a variety of data collection strategies that included semi-structured interviews, participant observation, a collaborative partnership, photovoice, focus group interviews,[65] and attendance at monthly CHWOI meetings via Zoom. Semi-structured interviews with CHWs comprised the bulk of the data. Interviews typically lasted 45 to 60 minutes and were audio-recorded and transcribed for data analysis. Participant demographics are presented in table 0.2.

Participant observation—in which I observed or directly participated in a variety of activities—also served as a primary data collection strategy (n < 300 hours). I earned a certification as a CHW, helped teach the CHW certification course with Lucía, and shadowed some of the participants (n = 3). Field notes were either handwritten and/or typed following each event for later data analysis.[66] While participant observation served as a primary data collection strategy, it was difficult[67] to collect data via this means. Thus, the findings related to client interactions derive mostly from semi-structured interviews with participants. Nonetheless, participant observation by attending certification courses, neighborhood tours with participants, Zoom meetings, and the

Table 0.2   Demographic Characteristics of the CHW Sample

Demographic Characteristics		N = 49
Age		
	18–30	12
	31–60	27
	61+	10
Sex		
	Male	10
	Female	39
Race/Ethnicity		
	White	16
	Black	8
	Biracial	1
	Latinx	24
Paid or Unpaid		
	Paid	34
	Unpaid (Volunteer)	5
	Both	10

few chances I shadowed CHWs all frame and inform the findings presented in this book.

Photovoice also served as a key methodology. In photovoice, a sample of participants is gathered who then take photographs related to a question, prompt, or a series of these.[68] The photographs are gathered and analyzed as a group. The researcher's role is diminished and rather serves solely as a discussion moderator. In this way, the participants' role is elevated as they are the data collectors and interpreters, who also co-construct meaning as they discuss each other's photographs. Photovoice serves as a social-justice-aligned methodology as it is grounded in feminist theory, empowerment education, and fosters critical consciousness.[69] This method also enhanced the participation and collaborative partnership between myself, Lucía, CHWOI, and the participants. Several photographs from the photovoice project appear, with permission, throughout this book.[70]

For this project, I adopted the "collaborative anthropology" framework, which is defined as a process that develops a long-term relationship between the researcher(s) and the community members that also expresses and meets the interests of all parties involved.[71] In line with this approach, I collaborated closely with Lucía who—through her extensive connections in the CHW movement and previous research—helped shape the project and serve as a key source of support.[72] Additionally, three participants reviewed earlier drafts of this manuscript and offered additional feedback and critique.[73] The collaborative framing of this project was an essential method in conducting research with CHWs. Anthropologists, scholars, and CHW organizations have also noted the need for collaborative approaches in research studies with these workers.[74] Lastly, the project detailed in this book was approved by the Institutional Review Board at the University of South Florida.

OVERVIEW OF CHAPTERS

In chapter 1, I explore the "moral economy of care" within which CHWs operate and how their caregiving is shaped by the political economic context in Indiana. I describe the characteristics of this moral economy, including the resources available, disparities faced in the communities that CHWs serve, state and federal policies affecting health and social services, and characterizations by participants of their commitment and connection to their clients and communities. I argue that, in order to fully understand the impact of CHWs in the pursuit of well-being and caregiving, it is essential to analyze and understand their moral drive and the connection CHWs maintain and cultivate with their communities and clients. Additionally, this chapter elucidates macro-level forces such as law, policy, and public sentiment and how these shape the ground-level experiences of CHWs and their communities.

Chapter 2 narrows the lens and arguments presented in the previous chapter. Here, I specifically analyze the CHW-client relationship within the framework of moral economy and assess the ways in which CHWs connect with clients and leverage various sociodemographic factors to motivate their clients to attain health and well-being. CHWs described the positive benefits of drawing on shared sociodemographic factors (e.g., race, class, gender, ethnicity, culture) to connect with clients in helping them become motivated to take control of their health and well-being. This chapter illustrates the various ways CHWs connect with and motivate their clients in addition to the challenges experienced in this relationship. I also assess how CHWs replicate the neoliberal approach to care found throughout the U.S. healthcare system, which frames the individual as being solely responsible for their health. I explore this issue and how CHWs mitigate this approach to care via advocacy and the steps they take to undermine the structural violence affecting their communities.

Chapter 3 explores the structural issues encountered by CHWs within the professional workforce including exclusion, confusion, and, at times, outright hostility from medical professionals. This lack of awareness has complicated and delayed the acceptance of CHWs within the professional workforce and has hindered their ability to aid clients adequately in the pursuit of well-being. Although CHWs have found greater acceptance in other states, in Indiana, CHWs were only beginning to be formally integrated during this study. I utilize the concept of professional citizenship to reveal the issues these workers encountered during professionalization and discuss the ramifications of this process. To facilitate their professional citizenship, a state-backed certification was developed for CHWs that would provide them with further legitimacy in addition to serving as a qualifier for Medicaid reimbursement for a designated set of CHW-specific services. I assess the positive and negative impacts of this certification as well as a variety of other professional barriers encountered by CHWs.

Building on the previous chapter, I analyze the boundaries that CHWs faced when aiding clients. I explore how their relative rejection and exclusion from the health and social services workforce placed many participants in a position in which they had to decide if they should remain within their scope of care (essentially, their designated responsibilities as a CHW) or go outside of this scope. While there is an overarching scope of care, CHWs may have additional boundaries designated by their employers and/or specific specialty trainings/positions (e.g., as doulas, midwives, medical interpreters, or diabetes educators). I demonstrate how participants grappled with deciding whether or not to cross boundaries and the ramifications of their choices. For some participants, going outside of these boundaries was justified by their obligation to provide care to someone in desperate need. Others believed that they could not cross certain boundaries due to professional reasons and/or personal beliefs and values.

Advocacy is a core role fulfilled by CHWs and serves to improve the overall well-being of their clients. In chapter 5, I argue that the advocacy performed by CHWs must be reconceptualized as a form of caregiving—especially as a means to improve health at the individual, organizational, community, and societal levels. By means of advocacy, CHWs play an essential role in addressing individual client needs. Such work fills gaps in the provision of care and addresses issues within organizations, the broader community, and within society to improve health outcomes. I also describe how CHWs in the study not only advocated for clients and their communities but also advocated to their own employers and to medical and social services professionals. Often they found themselves advocating for the legitimacy of their roles within the healthcare team as well as arguing against cutting social programs that positively impact their communities. Reconceptualizing advocacy as a form of caregiving offers further reason to enshrine it as a core role that enhances client health.

Given the stressful conditions CHWs find themselves in, chapter 6 reveals how these workers experience burnout and compassion fatigue. Few studies have explored the impact of burnout and insufficient self-care among CHWs. This chapter illuminates the causes of burnout and compassion fatigue in addition to revealing the steps taken by CHWs to avoid experiencing these professionally and emotionally deleterious conditions. I also assess the divisive strategy of "tough love" used by some as a form of self-care when dealing with difficult clients. Additionally, I analyze the professional needs of these workers and steps that can be taken, going forward, to diminish the frequency, severity, and effects of burnout and compassion fatigue. I also present several recommendations for addressing these conditions that current and potential employers may consider implementing.

I conclude by summarizing the key points and arguments made throughout the book regarding the moral economy of care of CHWs, the CHW-client relationship, the professional citizenship of these workers, boundaries and barriers to care, advocacy as a form of caregiving, and the impacts of burnout and the self-care practices of CHWs. In the Conclusion, I suggest avenues for future research and provide a variety of practical applications and recommendations. Furthermore, the findings presented in this book contribute to and complement an established, broader body of anthropological literature on medical paraprofessionals and auxiliary workers in health care.[75] Ultimately, the ethnographic findings presented in this book elucidate a complex and nuanced framing of the lived experiences of CHWs and present applicable findings that can significantly inform policy and advance the CHW movement.

NOTES

1. Structural violence is a concept introduced by Johan Galtung, defined as "the indirect violence built into repressive social orders creating enormous differences between potential and actual human self-realization" (Galtung 1975, 173). Structural violence is abstract in that it takes the forms of policies and laws and via political and social exclusion that inhibit and impede certain populations from equality and opportunity in a society.

2. See https://www.chicagotribune.com/suburbs/post-tribune/ct-ptb-east-chicago-one-year-later-st-0723-20170721-story.html.

3. See http://indianaindicators.org/dash/map.aspx.

4. APHA 2021.

5. All names of individuals and organizations are pseudonyms to protect identities.

6. "Client" was the preferred term utilized by participants in this project for individuals to whom CHWs provided care and services.

7. Medicare is a federal health insurance program for people aged 65 or older and may include others based on other eligibility criteria, for more information, see https://www.medicare.gov/what-medicare-covers/your-medicare-coverage-choices/whats-medicare.

8. See, e.g., Arvey et al. 2012, Deitrick et al. 2010, Encalada et al. 2019, Ingram et al. 2014, Katigbak et al. 2015, Nebeker et al. 2020, Pérez-Escamilla et al. 2015, Perry et al. 2014, Sabo et al. 2015, Shepard-Banigan et al. 2014, Valen et al. 2012.

9. See https://www.forbes.com/sites/richardlevick/2018/12/05/five-steps-to-heal-the-healthcare-workforce-shortage-crisis/#587b3d604aec.

10. Wasserman et al. 2019.

11. The name of this organization is a pseudonym.

12. APHA 2021.

13. Pérez and Martinez 2008, Perry et al. 2014.

14. Perry et al. 2014.

15. Pérez and Martinez 2008, Perry et al. 2014.

16. Pérez and Martinez 2008.

17. Ibid.

18. Ibid.

19. Ibid.

20. George et al. 2020, Ingram et al. 2020, Rosenthal et al. 2010.

21. U.S. Bureau of Labor Statistics 2018.

22. Perry et al. 2014.

23. Ibid.

24. Closser 2015, Maes 2017, Nading 2013.

25. Closser 2015, Maes 2015b, Maupin 2011, van de Ruit 2019.
26. Maupin 2011.
27. Zabiliūtė 2021.
28. See, e.g., Arvey et al. 2012, Cross-Barnet et al. 2018, Deitrick et al. 2010, Encalada et al. 2019, Ingram et al. 2014, Katigbak et al. 2015, Kreiger et al. 2011, Nebeker et al. 2020, Pérez-Escamilla et al. 2015, Perry et al. 2014, Ryabov 2014, Sabo et al. 2015, Shepard-Banigan et al. 2014, Valen et al. 2012, Viswanathan et al. 2010.
29. Cross-Barnet et al. 2018, Kreiger et al. 2011, Ryabov 2014, Viswanathan et al. 2010.
30. Bovbjerg et al. 2013, George et al. 2020, Katzen and Morgan 2014, Rosenthal et al. 2010.
31. This is known as Indiana as the "Healthy Indiana Plan 2.0," stylized as "HIP 2.0."
32. Groppe 2017.
33. Thompson 1971.
34. Scott 1976.
35. Thompson 1971: 79.
36. See, e.g., Bourgois 1998, Closser 2015; Fassin 2012, 2013; Horton 2015; Maes 2017; Nading 2013; Prince 2012.
37. Fassin 2012: 266.
38. Quesada et al. 2011: 341.
39. CHW Central 2017.
40. U.S. Department of Health and Human Services 2007.
41. Good et al. 2010: 177.
42. Logan 2021, 194.
43. U.S. Census Bureau 2019a.
44. Ibid.
45. American Immigration Council 2015, 2017.
46. Choi 2016, Puente 2007.
47. American Immigration Council 2017.
48. American Immigration Council 2015.
49. Pew Research Center 2016.
50. U.S. Census Bureau 2019b.
51. "Hoosier" is the demonym for people from Indiana, "Hoosier hospitality" is the well-known slogan that describes the state's residents' goodwill toward visitors.
52. Chavez et al. 2013.
53. Taylor et al. 2020.
54. America's Health Rankings 2020.
55. Indiana's public health funding in 2020 was $55 per capita (America's Health Rankings 2020).
56. Defined as "percentage of adults who reported their mental health was not good 14 or more days in the past 30 days" (America's Health Rankings 2020).
57. Defined as "percentage of adults who reported their physical health was not good 14 or more days in the past 30 days" (America's Health Rankings 2020).

58. America's Health Rankings 2020.

59. Ibid.

60. Indiana State Department of Health 2016.

61. Robert Wood Johnson Foundation 2018.

62. Ibid.

63. Ibid.

64. Ibid.

65. Three focus group interviews were conducted during the course of the study. The first was with a small group of CHWs who worked for a small employer and found it easiest to participate in the project together. This focus group utilized the same interview guide as done with the semi-structured interviews. The second focus group took place during the discussion of the photovoice photographs. The final focus group interview took place with several participants, in which I presented the initial findings from the research project. This served as an additional means to amplify the voices of the participants, refine the analysis of the data, and improve the internal validity of the study. This focus group provided a means to cross-check the findings gathered from "non-collaborative" methods (i.e., data gathered via semi-structured interviews and participant observation) and critically analyze my initial interpretations of the findings. This presentation to the participants helped to diminish any a priori assumptions I may have inserted into the findings during data analysis (Holmes and Castañeda 2014, 273). Finally, several participants reviewed initial drafts of this manuscript to offer additional feedback and critique.

66. All transcripts of the semi-structured interviews, focus group interview transcripts, and typed field notes were uploaded into MAXQDA (a qualitative data analysis program). All data were de-identified to protect the identities of participants and each were assigned a pseudonym. Some details were omitted to protect identities of participants. I drew on the use of grounded theory (Corbin and Strauss 2008) in order to identify emergent themes during data analysis.

67. Despite the acceptance from CHWs and their explanations to clients regarding my study, I felt my presence in these instances was detrimental to the interaction between the CHW and their client. Additionally, there were data collection restrictions due to IRB and Health Insurance Portability and Accountability Act (HIPAA) guidelines that limited my ability to conduct data collection in these interactions.

68. Wang and Burris 1997.

69. Gómez and Castañeda 2018, Mayfield-Johnson et al. 2014, Langhout 2014, Logan 2018, Wang 1999.

70. Although only a few studies had completed photovoice projects with CHWs (or other similarly titled medical paraprofessionals), they yielded in-depth and ethnographically rich data. See, e.g., Baquero et al. 2014, Mayfield-Johnson et al. 2015, Mitchell et al. 2005, O'Donovan et al. 2019, Musoke et al. 2020.

71. Bade and Martinez 2014.

72. I consulted with Lucía during the pilot research, while refining of the project design, developing research questions, deciding on semi-structured interview questions, during the data collection process, and the initial data analysis and write-up from her feedback and that of other CHWs. This collaborative approach ensured an elevated role for research participants, provided additional insights that I might not

have otherwise been afforded, and enhanced the internal validity of the findings. As a core factor of this collaboration, Lucía and the CHWOI organization made an exception in allowing me to train as a CHW in the certification class. This strengthened my understanding of the training of these workers and would also allow me to co-instruct certification courses with Lucía. She also correctly asserted that this would provide me with additional opportunities to study the material and training process of CHWs. In training as a CHW, I became embedded within the organization, provided me with detailed insights, and demonstrated my commitment to the organization and broader CHW movement. As such, I became a "participating" observer in tasks within the organization and during certification courses.

73. All findings were provided back to the partner organization in the form of peer-reviewed articles, two policy briefs (including one coauthored with Lucía), an executive summary of the primary research findings, and providing the photovoice photographs (with written consent) of the participants for CHWOI to utilize in their endeavors.

74. C3 2018; Maes et al. 2014; Nebeker et al. 2015, 2020.

75. See, e.g., Backe 2018, Besterman-Dahan et al. 2014, Brodwin 2008, Buch 2013, Contreras et al. 2012, Davis-Floyd and Davis 1996, Deitrick et al. 2010, Fisher 2018a., Getrich et al. 2007, Price 2014, Stevenson 2014, Zigon 2011.

Chapter 1

"There Is Hope Out There"

Community Health Workers and the Moral Economy of Care

"What motivates me is that I was in their place," Maricela recounted to me during our conversation. A middle-aged Latinx woman, Maricela came to northeastern Indiana from Puerto Rico in the early 2000s. Two key moments changed the career trajectory that Maricela had envisioned for herself. Although she earned a degree in accounting by the mid-2000s and had planned to work "in front of a computer and do paperwork," Maricela had continued her employment as an assistant to a Spanish instructor at a local school. Maricela explained to me that it was this instructor who originally pushed her to think about a future meeting her community's needs. "I'm no tutor and no teacher," Maricela remarked to her boss. Remaining unconvinced by Maricela's words, her boss stated, "I see it in you. You are. You have so much knowledge. I see you working in groups, and I see how you manage that kind of pressure and structure. So, I think that you will be perfect for this [for serving the community]."

This conversation left a lasting impression on Maricela but it was another event that finally prompted her into this line of work. She remarked to me, "Once I needed an interpreter, I needed a health navigator, I needed someone that could teach me how to take care of my ear situation. I have an ENT [ears, nose, and throat] health condition. Someone took their time to sit down with me and it wasn't a medical professional. It was someone in the community." For Maricela, the aid she received from this community member in her time of need deeply shaped her desire to look into ways to help the community. She added, "Gosh, if it benefitted me, I imagine it could benefit others also." Maricela soon found an avenue into work as a medical interpreter when a grant-funded position was made available. Maricela applied and was soon on her way to Indianapolis for a week to earn her certification as a medical interpreter. However, aside from her duties as a medical interpreter, Maricela also functioned in the role of a CHW, aiding clients with other health and social service needs outside the clinic. She explained, "And that I loved. I got to work with the community one-on-one and I've learned my boundaries, but as a community health worker, you are that [a translator] plus anything else you can assist your client with."

Although each participant had a unique story about why they became a CHW, their stories parallel Maricela's experience: a deep connection to the community, to sharing their experience via outreach, a commitment to social justice, the satisfaction of inspiring others to become empowered with regard to their own well-being, and paying it forward. Such emotions, morals, values, motivations, and obligations elucidate the nuances of the lived experience of CHWs via the lens of moral economy. Dider Fassin defines this framework as "the production, distribution, circulation, and utilization of moral sentiments, emotions, and values, norms and obligation in the social space."[1] Fassin[2] further emphasizes that moral economy must be understood within the current social and historical context. For CHWs, this underscores the need to understand the political economy in which they function (e.g., political rhetoric, state and federal laws, the history of the CHW workforce). Analyzing the lived experiences of CHWs through this framework elicits insights into the constellation of factors that motivate CHWs, how they function, how they structure their relationships, and what drives them to make positive changes in their communities.

Anthropological studies utilizing the lens of moral economy have revealed the nuances within the relationships between CHWs and their communities, employers, the broader society, and have illuminated, in particular, how these workers structure their motivations and caregiving.[3] These studies have identified the structural forces that shape the moral economy of CHWs and the value of understanding the motivations, morals, values, and approaches CHWs take in fostering relationships with their communities, employers, and other stakeholders. Maes[4] and Closser[5] drew on moral economy in order to understand how relationships are constructed between employers and nongovernmental organizations (NGOs) in terms of how they conceptualize CHWs. Employers and NGOs understand CHWs as individuals motivated as altruistic volunteers.[6] This conception directly impacts the remuneration of CHWs, leading to some being unpaid or receiving meager salaries. CHWs in these studies described the need for increased pay in order to survive. While they truly wanted to help their communities, they still considered their work worthy of remuneration. These examples illustrate some of the insights into the work of CHWs that can be derived by drawing on moral economy. In addition to their altruistic motivations and their desire to earn a living, it is apparent that a wide range of other factors motivate these workers, including morals, religion, and culture.[7]

This chapter explores how CHWs in Indiana engage in a *moral economy of care*. I adopt a similar framing as described by Watters,[8] who defines a moral economy of care in relation to the provision of resources and services to refugees, asylum seekers, and undocumented migrants in Europe based on societal conceptions of legitimacy and illegitimacy—essentially how care and provision of services are determined based on the deservingness of the recipient. In the case of CHWs in Indiana, I define this moral economy of care as the landscape in which CHWs in Indiana function, the morals, values, and obligations that make their caregiving unique and the forces that complicate their ability to provide care. This moral economy of care is shaped by structural factors that include laws, policies, ethics, morals, and conceptions of deservingness, which are in turn affected by the political climate (such as anti-immigrant rhetoric and punitive laws and policies against immigrants, Black, Indigenous, Asian populations; and populations experiencing homelessness, mental health disorders, and/or substance use disorder). The overarching factors and the variety of sentiments circulating at the ground level affect and mold relationships between CHWs, clients, and other stakeholders (e.g., medical, public health and social service professionals, policy-makers, employers). This chapter focuses on how the broader political climate—both at the national and state levels including laws, public health policy, and public sentiment—shapes the moral economy of care of CHWs and their communities in Indiana. These macro-level forces enact boundaries that directly impact the ability of these workers to form relationships, effectively perform their roles as CHWs, and shape the overall well-being of their clients.

Analyzing and understanding how these forces shape the moral economy of care is crucial to elucidating their effects on the micro-level interactions between CHWs, clients, and other stakeholders. The moral economy of care in Indiana comprises a constellation of moving factors, examined here, that include access to care, resources directly or indirectly related to health and well-being, the morals of CHWs and of people in the political and social worlds in which CHWs operate, and federal and state policies and laws. The structural vulnerability of clients is also assessed and varies depending on sociodemographic factors (e.g., race, ethnicity, language, legal status), which can present additional barriers to accessing care and resources. This moral economy is complex and fluctuating, depending on laws, policy, structural vulnerability, and the precarious position of CHWs within the broader workforce.

"THE NEEDS ARE GREAT": STRUCTURAL FACTORS
SHAPING THE MORAL ECONOMY OF CARE

I spent a day meeting with CHWs at a small, community-based organization in a large, northeastern Indiana city in July 2017. Even in the early morning hours as I arrived in the city, it was hot, and the humidity was rising. This city has a significant Black population, and many residents are affected by various social determinants of health, including lack of financial capital, public transportation, access to care, safe outdoor environments, housing, and food. These social determinants of health not only serve as barriers to healthy living but also directly lead to increased morbidity and mortality.[9] Additionally, these determinants are largely perpetuated by overarching structural forces such as racist and discriminatory policies that place resources out of reach and communities in deleterious situations. These determinants are well understood by CHWs, as many participants experience(d) them and can help clients find ways to circumvent them.

During my visit, I met with Beverly, a middle-aged, Black woman who has more than a decade of experience as a CHW. Her connection to the community is evident. Though possessing a no-nonsense kind of attitude, she is kind-hearted and has a deep passion for improving the well-being of her clients and the broader community. "Where we are a located, we see the needs are great and that people are feeling helpless and hopeless. . . . We can break down the barrier," Beverly spoke candidly to me regarding the obstacles facing her community. She simultaneously noted how structural forces crushingly shape her clients' experiences and how CHWs can play an important role in addressing these issues. She noted that CHWs can change clients' perspectives by "letting them know that there is hope out there and we [CHWs] are here to help you in any way that we can. People sometimes feel so defeated that they just give up and they pursue it no longer." Beverly explained how the aid provided to clients makes all the difference, stating, "And then a word is said, or somebody's done something that they think, 'Ok, one more time. I'm going to try one more time and see where it goes.'"

This connection CHWs felt to their community was foundational. Not all relationships with clients were successful, but dedication to the community and knowledge of the challenges experienced by clients (often, first-hand knowledge) were important sources for CHWs to draw on as they provided care. This was especially true when it came to addressing the impact of the aforementioned social determinants of health and how structural violence affects their communities. As Beverly noted, sometimes one action by or word from a CHW changes the perspective of the client and leads them to persevere. She also acknowledged her own structural vulnerability, adding "I mean, it's compassion for people because but by the grace of God, we could be in the positions that we find people in." In this way, CHWs through their approach to caregiving address and circumvent these determinants.

As discussed in the Introduction, Indiana has consistently ranked in the bottom third of states in terms of overall health. One structural factor affecting this poor performance is the lack of investment in public health. Public health spending, at $55[10] per capita in Indiana, is an indicator of and correlates with a variety of chronic illnesses and health outcomes[11]—health issues that CHWs can positively address.[12] This lack of investment in public health results in the significant health issues detailed in the Introduction. The resulting dearth of preventative measures can result in deadly and costly chronic diseases such as diabetes, cancer, and heart disease. Investing in the CHW workforce is one means to help individuals improve their health, practice risk reduction, and access and benefit from health education. The aid in access to care provided by CHWs can help stop these issues or, at least, reduce their severity. Unfortunately, a variety of laws and policies complicate the moral economy of care.

LAWS AND POLICIES

Laws and policies influence the moral economy of care, and facilitate the structural violence inflicted on communities, and create structural vulnerabilities to which specific populations (e.g., immigrant, Black, Latinx, etc.) are exposed. These same forces exert strain on CHWs too. Iain Wilkinson and Arthur Kleinman address the structural vulnerability of care workers, noting that they are "among the lowest paid in our economy, have little political power, and occupy positions of low social status" and "tend to be women from lower socioeconomic groups . . . classified as immigrants or people of color."[13] As noted previously, most CHWs in this study and throughout much of the world are women of color and continue to experience structural vulnerability in spite of their position and ability to navigate a landscape of resources and serve as caregivers. However, while experiencing structural vulnerability affects the CHWs, they draw on this shared experience with clients in helping to motivate them, a topic I detail later in this chapter.

Several federal laws shape the moral economy of care in Indiana. The Patient Protection and Affordable Care Act (ACA) of 2010 was a landmark piece of legislation in the United States that provided insurance to a significant portion of the U.S. population. Many others found insurance through the Medicaid expansion that followed. This law provided symbolic steps forward by recognizing CHWs by name as well as proposing funding streams for CHW programs.[14] Additionally, the sections of the ACA that cover these workers were pivotal in that they were written by a variety of stakeholders including prominent CHWs. In other words, CHWs themselves helped craft this portion of the legislation.[15] While the funding allotted to the CHW grants was cut during the markup of the bill, the law retained verbiage related to CHWs, thereby helping to name brand the position and provide further recognition.[16] These workers are recognized in multiple sections of the ACA, which noted opportunities for CHWs in several areas, including health education centers (AHECs); hospital admission reduction, patient-centered medical homes (PCMH) and community health teams; maternal, infant, and early childhood home visiting programs (MIECHV); hospital community benefits; and grants to promote the community health workforce.[17] Overall, recognition of CHWs in the ACA underscores their potential.

Other federal laws and programs have also produced impacts on the moral economy of care for CHWs and their clients. The Health Insurance Portability and Accountability Act (HIPAA) of 1996 significantly altered the handling of patient data and privacy in order to provide further protections for patient medical information. This law shapes the care CHWs can provide and hinders some from fully aiding clients. Some participants in this study noted how cultural norms related to privacy and familial care can clash with this law (see chapter 4 for further details). Medicaid—a joint federal and state health insurance program—impacts the moral economy of care as many of the clients of CHWs receive insurance through this program and thereby access health care and resources. CHWs must also be aware of Medicaid and how it functions in Indiana and potentially assist qualifying clients in signing up. The program also became pivotal to CHWs in Indiana because a CHW-specific set of billable services reimbursable through Medicaid was developed for the employers of these workers (see chapter 3).

In addition to being affected by federal laws and programs, the care provided by CHWs is shaped by other forces, including the national CHW code of ethics, scopes of care (e.g., the scope of care provided in the CHW certification course, employer-designated responsibilities), and additional organizational and/or employer guidelines and rules regarding care. These various forces enact boundaries related to the care and caregiving activities that can be provided by CHWs. At times, these boundaries come into conflict with the morals and motivations of the workers. As I describe in this chapter and in chapter 4, some participants remained dedicated to strictly following their scope of care while others challenged and crossed these boundaries.

Overall, the moral economy of care is shaped through federal laws and programs, codes of ethics, and scopes of care, and regulated via certification and further trainings provided by employers and other organizations. CHWs had to be aware of these laws, policies, and scopes of care in order to be compliant with any regulations and employer policies while providing care. However, these could be mitigated by the moral economy of care in pursuit of providing the needed services and care to clients—illustrated by how, at times, these rules and regulations could conflict with the morals and motivations of CHWs. It was up to the individual CHW to stay within or go outside the scope of care in order to provide services or resources needed by the client.

Under the context of these laws, policies, and regulations, maintaining a connection to the community and building relationships with clients was essential. In the breakroom of her community-based organization, Beverly emphasized how CHWs' in-the-community approach to care provides a unique lens from which to offer health education and other services. She told me, "Because health education is what we do . . . we are just out in the community. We are in the mud with the people. We are right there in the trenches with them. Helping them, letting them know that we understand a lot about what they are going through." In emphasizing how CHWs are in the trenches, Beverly recognizes the power of the shared lived experience with their clients, which serves as an anchor joining CHWs to their clients and the broader community within the moral economy of care. She continued, "We are out there talking to people and listening to them. . . . When people really feel that you have a sense of really caring about them and their well-being, they tend to open up a little bit more to you." This demonstrates how the relationships maintained by CHWs are pivotal to improving health outcomes and underscoring the value of CHWs working within the communities they come from. Beverly concluded, "So, you are really a community health worker almost all the time . . . you are just with people where they are."

Being part of the community, relating similar experiences, and emphasizing that CHWs "understand a lot about what they are going through" were vital components that (1) establish CHWs as a unique component of the health and social services workforce and (2) establish trusting and committed relationships within the moral economy of care. These workers are impacted at the ground level as structural forces in the form of laws, policies, and regulations that shape structural vulnerability and the accessibility of care and resources for clients and communities. CHWs drew on their moral obligations to their communities and operationalized trust and commitment to build relationships and lead clients to improved health and well-being. Moreover, due to their understanding of the various ways structural forces shape care at the ground level, they are able to establish profound relationships with their clients. Lastly, some CHWs provided essential input—based on this knowledge and lived experience—to local, state, and federal legislators and to their managers that helped to inform, adjust, and potentially change policies and laws to better facilitate caregiving.

ATYPICAL AS TYPICAL: THE WORK LIFE OF CHWS

When I met with CHWs, I'd ask them to describe a "typical" day. Normally, when I'd ask this question, the answers would be similar to those of Beverly and her supervisor. I met with Beverly's boss, a middle-aged Black woman named Marcia who is also a CHW and executive director of a community-based health organization. I asked her to describe her typical day. She responded, "Typical?! No two [days] are the exactly the same . . . you don't know what's going to happen any given moment." The unpredictability of CHWs' workdays is a direct result of the macro-level forces (e.g., laws, policy, structural violence) and their impacts on the communities served by CHWs. Other factors that shaped their workday included lack of professional incorporation and the natural variability that occurs when conducting outreach and providing services in the community.

Beverly also echoed these sentiments, explaining that she could have planned out her entire workday only for her plans to be thrown completely off due to walk-ins, unexpected issues that arose during outreach, and other impromptu events. Beverly explained that the habitual lack of consistency could lead to frustration but that being flexible was a skill requisite for CHWs, needed if they were to maintain calmness and keep the needs of the client at the core. She explained,

> And if you're not flexible it can really make you a little batty. You can get a bit frustrated too. . . . People need things . . . and you have to stop what you're doing and kind of investigate because you can feel the urgency in their voice that they need something. And if we can help them, you've got to drop what you're doing and see if you can help them.

The lack of consistency in the moral economy of care challenged participants to plan for the unexpected as best they could and to respond flexibly to the issues they encountered. Some participants noted that flexibility must be an innate quality possessed by CHWs and those who wish to become CHWs. This character trait was also important given the disparate and siloed nature of resources, detailed in the next section. Furthermore, several participants noted that flexibility also functions as a form of self-care in and of itself (a topic I elaborate on chapter 6). Possessing this mindset was crucial to not becoming overwhelmed throughout the course of a day.

Aside from needing to remain flexible and to expect the unexpected, participants identified that regular outreach within the community was a core component of their daily work routine. This public presence within the community served as an important pillar that reinforced their position within the moral economy of care, as it built rapport and trust through direct engagement with community members. As a unique role of CHWs, one that sets them apart from biomedical professionals (e.g., nurses, doctors, medical assistants), this outreach also serves to address a gap in care by helping clients with issues they encountered on a daily basis—often outside the realm of the clinic. This type of extensive outreach is not typical for medical doctors and other professionals, who do not regularly engage with the community outside of the hospital, clinic, or community-based organizations.

Causes versus Symptoms and "Journeying" with Clients

Almost two years later, I conducted a follow-up interview with Beverly. She candidly summed up her view of how CHWs approach clients, as opposed to biomedical professionals: "You're in the trenches with them so you understand it [the lives of the patients]. The doctors are on top of the hill, while you are in the valley. You're [the patients] like cattle, they're [the doctors] just pushing you through." Beverly emphasized that it is through commitment to clients and the community via direct engagement that CHWs uncover the health and social needs. She asserted, "Well, CHWs take that time to understand their [client's] issues. CHWs will ask, '*Why* are you sick?' . . . doctors only want to know the *symptoms*. They don't want to know the *causes*."

Beverly's example highlights a core component of the CHW model—that these workers focus on the *causes* and not simply the *symptoms* of deleterious conditions. Furthermore, this profound level of understanding and shared experience are powerful connectors between CHWs and clients. Via their outreach within the community, CHWs identify issues missed within the doctor's appointment—primarily the social determinants of health that impede or restrict the ability of clients to adhere to treatment plans and/or achieve overall well-being. Other participants described their work as being on a "journey" with their clients.

In early 2018, I met with Alisha, a CHW with 19 years of experience who identifies as biracial. I asked her to explain how she approaches her work with clients, which she described as "journey[ing] with people." Alisha asserted that in sharing in her clients' journeys, she learned of their needs, challenges, and appropriate resources to provide them with. Echoing Beverly, Alisha described how her work spanned more than just identifying the health needs of her clients: "I was the eyes and ears for that [client's] doctor—to say, 'Well, guess what, I went to the home and they're actually hoarders and they have their needles everywhere, and we need to get some other services in there.'" As a result, Alisha navigated both the health and social needs of clients. As she explained, "So, not only was I connecting with the health side of it, I was also connected with the social service side of it, making sure that the patient was as healthy as they could possibly be."

Her example demonstrates that community outreach and developing a relationship with the client outside the clinic is key to understanding issues in the community and in the home in addition to providing additional services that might be needed. And while some CHWs are employed in clinics or hospitals, their ability to directly engage the community "in the trenches" is a vital component of their daily work life, enabling them to remain part of the moral economy of care.

Religiosity, Compassion, and Understanding

Participants in this study described a variety of other qualities and skills as being crucial to CHWs, enabling them to navigate effectively within the moral economy of care. While I elaborate on these topics in the subsequent chapter, it is worthwhile to note here that these skills and systems of belief were important for CHWs to remain resilient in the face of structural violence and racism. For example, CHWs described drawing inspiration from either their religion, altruism, and/or moral standpoint to guide them in their work. Several participants were motivated by religious conviction and referenced God as a primary source of motivation and self-care within the moral economy of care. However, it is important to note that there was a distinct line here that CHWs did not cross: they did not proselytize or persecute clients for supposed religious or moral failings related to their health issues, well-being, gender identity, or sexual orientation. If a CHW was feeling somehow morally challenged by a client, they would identify another CHW or service provider who could help this client.[18] For participants, drawing on these belief systems reinforced their approach, helping them to remain resolutely focused on keeping the health and well-being of the client at the center of their caregiving.

This religiosity served as an impetus for the work of many participants and as a source of internal strength and motivation. Their religiosity reinforced their commitment and moral obligation to their clients and the community, thereby fortifying their own participation and belongingness within the moral economy of care. This religious commitment to providing access to care and resources, circumventing the social determinants of health, and dedication to social justice and helping clients improve their overall well-being stood, ironically, in contrast to the domineering religio-conservative nature of Indiana's politics. These conservative politics are practiced by politicians who espouse their "religious" convictions but instead deny care and resources to those most in need through laws, policies, and failure to fund public health in the state. CHWs, on the other hand, viewed themselves as "doing God's work" through providing access to care, remaining steadfast in their commitment to social justice, and improving the overall well-being of their clients.

Other participants described being motivated by a sense of compassion and understanding of their clients and wanting them to live their lives to their fullest and healthiest. During the photovoice component of the overall project, I met Mark—a White paramedic and CHW in his late 30s, who was part of a specialized unit that makes house visits to patients who had been identified by his employing organization as "repeat visitors" to emergency departments at hospitals in Indianapolis (i.e., patients who presented at the emergency departments multiple times for nonemergency conditions or for emergencies, such as severe hypoglycemia,[19] resulting from untreated chronic conditions). His unit was created to meet the needs of these repeat visitors, to address these needs *before* they reached emergency levels, to offer preventative care, and to connect these individuals with other health and social service needs.

To better understand how to work within the community and conduct public outreach, Mark and his fellow paramedics completed the CHW certification course. Mark submitted a photograph to encapsulate his experience as a CHW and, as a caption to his photograph, composed a prose poem about how he views his outreach within the community (see figure 1.1).

Mark's notion that being a CHW is equivalent to "opportunity" rather than a "duty" underscores a unique viewpoint common to those who do this job. His poem and photo collage highlight how outreach serves as an opportunity to help those in his community—especially those who are missed or excluded from biomedicine. The opening of the door provides an opportunity for the CHW to extend health care—through building and fostering a relationship within the moral economy of care. This concept recalls Beverly's comment about how a simple word can cause someone to say, "Ok, one more time. I'm going to try one more time and see where it goes."

Ultimately, the quotidian work life of CHWs is one marked by uncertainty and a need to maintain flexibility. The overarching environment made up of laws, policies, and health disparities indelibly shapes this uncertainty and enacts boundaries and barriers affecting the caregiving of these workers. Experience and flexibility allowed participants to prepare themselves mentally for unpredictable and constant unknowns. This mental preparation also served as a coping mechanism for CHWs to help them through their workdays. Furthermore, many participants drew on religion and/or a moral obligation to their clients and communities, thereby cementing their role within the moral economy of care. These factors largely contributed to the foundation for participants to engage in this work and navigate the complex economy of resources and potential boundaries created by the social determinants of health.

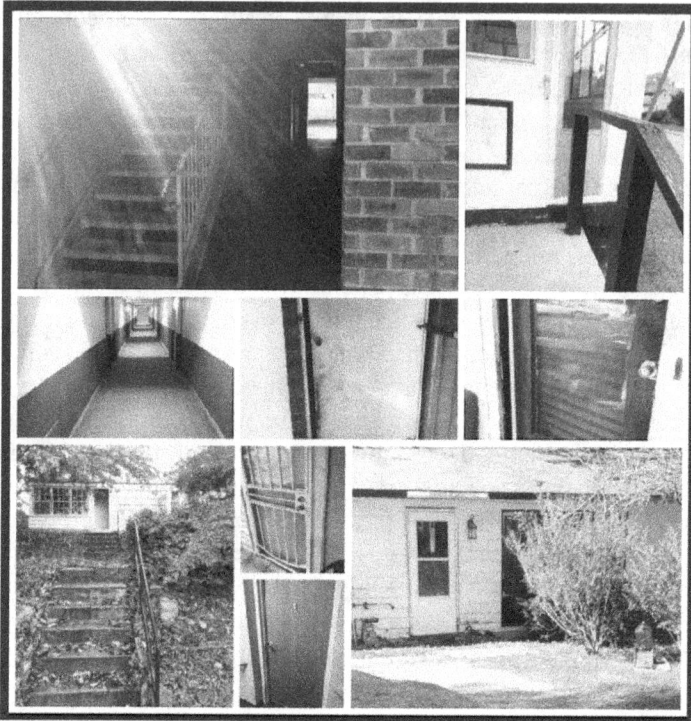

Figure 1.1   "Each of these doors, stairs, and halls have afforded me an opportunity . . . to meet a neighbor in need, in need of something, something that is always different, different but enlightening. Regardless of who is behind that door, up those stairs, or down the hall, these doors, stairs, and halls are thresholds to new relationships, steps to stronger communities and paths to healthier neighbors. Being a community health worker is not a duty, it is an opportunity to open closed doors, lift people to new heights, and brighten dimly lit halls—just like these doors, stairs, and halls have afforded me an opportunity." *Source:* Photo by Mark (Pseudonym).

EXTENDING OR SOFTENING THE MEDICAL GAZE?

CHWs encounter a variety of structural issues within communities and their outreach addresses a significant gap in the provision of care in the United States. Their day-to-day interactions within the community, traveling with clients, visiting their homes, and developing relationships can be viewed as extending the authority of medical professional, that is, the medical gaze,[20] from the medical appointment to the home environment. However, participants described being on the side of the client and assessing their needs, identifying barriers related to the social determinants of health, and aiding clients circumvent these challenges. Thus, CHWs do more than extend an authoritative medical gaze into their clients' lives; they soften it through their own lens of compassion, understanding, and advocacy.

This concept is encapsulated in the work of anthropologist Alex Nading[21] who assessed how *brigadistas* (CHWs) in Nicaragua served to biomedically "discipline" their neighbors to participate in public-health-mandated behavioral changes in order to mitigate the spread of mosquito-borne disease. At the same time, however, these brigadistas adopted a compassionate approach to their work—participating in a balancing act within this moral economy, including both their work obligations and their relationships with individuals in the community. Nading's analysis of the moral economy of medical citizenship experienced by CHWs highlights two reified conceptions of these workers. Public health and anthropological scholars have examined how these workers often become reified as either "extension agents" (of biomedicine) or "agents of change," specifically as described by Colvin and Swartz.[22] CHWs, however, often straddle between these two roles in a precarious balancing act in which they must, as detailed by Nading, maintain work obligations while also preserving their unique role in the moral economy of care by serving the community and individual clients.

CHWs in Indiana likewise straddled this liminal space. For example, participants noted having to carry out this balancing act to help clients adhere to a prescribed biomedical treatment plan, which could prove challenging for many due to financial barriers or lack of understanding. Patients who did not adhere to this plan risked being labeled as "noncompliant." Thus CHWs had to draw on their knowledge, compassion, trusted relationships, and shared lived experiences to aid clients in adhering to the prescribed biomedical treatments. Echoing the thoughts of other participants, Valeria, a CHW, explained that medical professionals might not take the time to explain how to carry out a treatment plan. Often, Valeria asserted, they will simply *tell* patients to follow a treatment plan instead of *showing* them how to carry it out. Although CHWs extend the medical gaze, their commitment to the community reinforces their belongingness and the patient's deservingness of care within the healthcare system, thereby promoting compassion and demonstrating the necessary steps to help clients attain well-being.

CHWs also soften the medical gaze through the practice of witnessing. This practice emphasizes a nonjudgmental approach to care, acknowledging the life of the patient, and focuses attention on how care is provided to and for the patient.[23] Davenport[24] explored the impact of this practice on medical students in training who were volunteers at a student-run clinic for individuals experiencing homelessness. Witnessing, Davenport, contends, "is also seen as a way to counter the symbolic violence of the medical gaze."[25] In their practice of relationship-building, compassion, and advocacy for their client, CHWs employ this same mode of care within the moral economy of care. As a result, CHWs subvert the medical gaze through witnessing and thereby serving as a source of support, understanding, and advocacy for their communities and clients.

Witnessing, as described by participants in this study, served as an important component in the repertoire of services and roles fulfilled by CHWs in order to soften and upend the medical gaze and biomedical approach. Additionally, this practice allowed these workers to understand the lives of their clients and identify social determinants of health that impeded their ability to improve their well-being. Building, maintaining, and reinforcing their relationships and maintaining a presence within their respective communities aided CHWs in becoming visible and trusted community members who could unlock opportunities, resources, and improve community and client health.

The medical gaze intimately structures the experience of the clients of CHWs in the biomedical realm and, in turn, can negatively affect the motivation and ability to adhere to treatment plans in structurally vulnerable populations. Experiencing this gaze affects how clients interact with and navigate the moral economy of care. CHWs must balance extending the reach of the medical gaze with being a compassionate neighbor.[26] Nevertheless, CHWs' ability to be successful in this balancing act is also affected by their ability to draw on resources within the moral economy of care.

"LIKE AN OCTOPUS": CHWS AND THE LANDSCAPE OF RESOURCES

Resources are a crucial element shaping the moral economy of care within which CHWs operate. Being knowledgeable not only about what resources are available but also which clients qualify for them was essential. These resources were numerous and varied. They included bus passes, diapers, eyeglasses, pill organizers, and food pantries and other organizations that CHWs could send clients to for various necessities. In my conversations with Mark, he emphasized that it was not only important for CHWs to maintain and curate this knowledge but also to navigate these resources effectively with clients. He stated, "It's about resources too, but if you don't know how to communicate those to your clients or how to navigate or utilize them, then you are ineffective, and you won't succeed as a CHW, and neither will your patients." Here, Mark not only highlighted a potential breakdown in the CHW-client relationship if the CHW is unable to help a client access resources but also underscored a breakdown in the moral economy of care. Failing as a CHW not only has implications for the individual client but could produce wider repercussions within the community—as clients could potentially be deprived of needed resources and services, become distrustful of CHWs, and share this experience with others.[27] Negative emotions and distrust could poison relationships between the CHW and the community.

In spite of the potential pitfalls, CHWs generally spoke positively of a wide variety of available resources. Often, those who worked in larger cities had easier access to a wider variety of resources. And despite the siloed nature of many of these resources, CHWs described weaving together these disparate assets to the benefit of their clients. In my conversation with Leticia, a middle-aged Latinx woman and a CHW with 11 years of experience now working primarily in the development of policy related to CHWs, she conceptualized CHWs as "connectors." Leticia mentioned how many health and social service providers—hospitals, community centers, and other organizations—are typically siloed. However, given that CHWs are out in the community and engage with these various stakeholders, these workers can pull together this disjointed landscape of resources and effectively connect clients to aid. Other participants also described CHWs similarly. Martha, a CHW also with 11 years of experience, explained how these workers are "someone [who's] like an octopus. They can take an arm and reach out anywhere and pull whatever the needs are because they know that community well and they know how to help that client and their clients trust them because it is someone I can identify with or the clients and community members can identify with."

Participants also spoke to their knowledge of the landscape of resources and how they had to serve as a "repository" of knowledge—as Martha asserted, "And that's where the CHW becomes valuable because each of our CHWs is like a repository. If it's something you need and it's not here, where else can I send you or refer you to? So that is where CHWs have to be like a little repository of what's going on around the whole state pretty much." Possessing this knowledge and actively working to build upon it were essential tasks for CHWs in order to for them to navigate effectively the moral economy of care and provide clients with the best possible services and resources. For many CHWs, it was entirely up to them to be aware of the plenitude of resources, their availability based on client qualifications, and how to draw on them effectively to achieve the maximum impact on the client's well-being.

However, participants noted a number of frustrations they were used to encountering when trying to access disparate and siloed resources for their clients. These frustrations included (1) the seemingly sudden appearance and disappearance of resources and aid organizations, (2) the lack of access due to the legal status of the client, (3) the lack of availability of a resource in one municipality or county of a resource easily available in another, and (4) the lack of a central database of available resources, much less one that is thorough and constantly updated. This issue was also discussed during the photovoice portion of the project. Isabella, a Latinx CHW in her mid-30s, came across an interesting scene within her community one day. She captured in a photograph this odd arrangement of discarded items that included two boots, a day planner, two toothbrushes, and a tube of toothpaste (see figure 1.2). She used this photograph in response to the prompt, "What is a challenge you have overcome as a CHW?"

After Isabella showed her photograph during the group discussion, the other participants joked that Isabella's photography almost resembled one of a crime scene that needed a forensic analysis. Jokes aside, Isabella further extrapolated on her photograph and caption:

> That's when self-doubt comes in. You know, you don't feel like you have the right tools or skills to help your client and you doubt yourself because you see a mess. You see all of this and you're like, "Oh no, I don't know if I can help them!" But in the depth of your heart, you know that you feel like you have to. You have to be there. You have to be there and consider that maybe just being present is part of putting the puzzle pieces together.

Isabella's photograph is a visual metaphor. The work of the CHW is one involving puzzle pieces—resources, organizations, or social determinants of

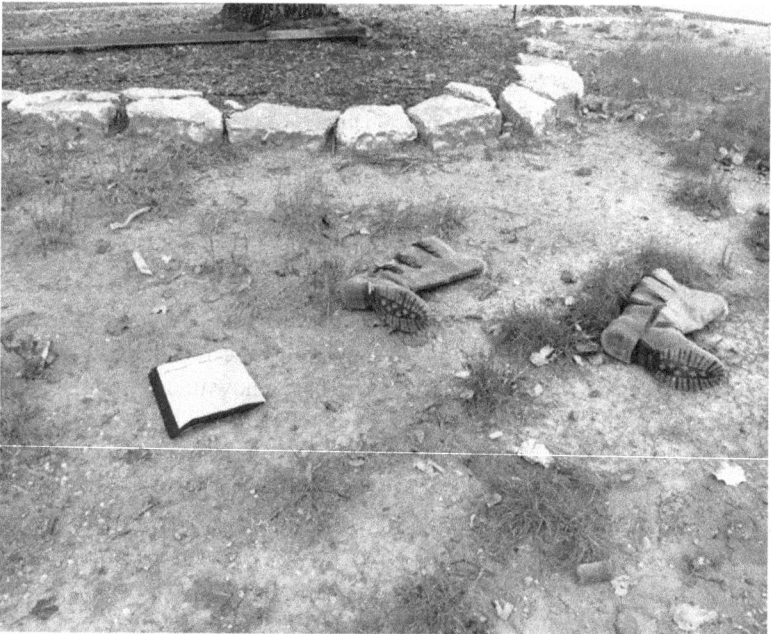

Figure 1.2 "Many times you may be apprehensive about what you see and doubt whether or not you have the ability to help put the puzzle pieces together." *Source:* Photo by Isabella (Pseudonym).

health—that CHWs must put together and arrange in the best way possible for the client. In this way, the CHW's presence within the moral economy of care serves as a critical factor in caregiving. Isabella's photograph also captures the disparate nature of siloed resources in Indiana, with the CHW serving as the facilitator between clients and these disparate resources. As Isabella notes, being present and assessing the situation helps to put the puzzle together.

Ultimately, the broader environment contains a variety of resources for CHWs to draw upon. These resources intimately shape the moral economy of care but can be impacted by lack of funding, availability, or qualifications (e.g., legal status) of clients to access them. It was largely the responsibility of the CHW to be aware of the resources in their local community and guide clients to each of these. While participants generally described a myriad of resources they could access for clients, significant challenges were present as a result of broader, structural forces.

CHALLENGES IN NAVIGATING
THE MORAL ECONOMY OF CARE

CHWs encountered a wide range of challenges, frustrations, and barriers within the moral economy of care in Indiana. Challenges included specific issues encountered by clients, community issues, challenges working with doctors and other professionals, and broader structural issues (e.g., provision of resources, client qualifications for access to care, and policies and laws that deny access to care/resources to particular populations).[28] Although participants often overcame these structural forces, at other times they were unable to or at least encountered significant barriers that could harm the well-being of the client due to being unable to provide care or resources.

Access to Resources

While it was beneficial for participants to be knowledgeable about the available resources, this value of having the right kind of knowledge also highlights a challenge within the moral economy. As noted earlier, CHWs described how some resources could seemingly be present one day and gone the next day. Organizations that provided resources and/or services in the community that participants relied on were crucial. But if funding could not be sustained, an organization and its resources could quickly be gone. In other instances, resources and their provision could differ dramatically between neighboring counties and even between neighboring cities. Participant CHWs also described finding resources new to them that had nonetheless existed for some time or discovering, too late, resources that could have been useful to clients. It was for these very reasons that having a central database or some physical or digital location that lists all of the resources available is necessary but also difficult to maintain. As a result of the lack of such an accessible and thorough database, CHWs were tasked with learning about the resources solely from first-hand experience, from their colleagues, from information numbers (such as 4-1-1), or from clients.

Participants also described still more challenges that their clients faced in accessing resources. In June 2017, I met with a CHW named Jane, a middle-aged White woman with six years of experience. Jane worked in north central Indiana and specialized in aiding clients with mental health disorders. Her clients lived in rural areas in this region and experienced unique issues compared to those in more urban settings. Jane explained that too often there is an assumption that everyone in the society has the same level of access to health care and other resources (e.g., transportation, internet access, a computer, a smartphone, etc.). "It just boils down to [the fact that] there needs to be more resources available, and people need to be able to access [them]. A lot of the clients don't have regular access to technology." Even though they might be able to access such resources in their community, she noted that these are not always available. She continued, "If they don't have a phone, how are they going to have a computer, or the internet? How are they going to have a way to get to the library? The library is not always open 24 hours a day to use a computer. If you don't have a library card or you have fines on your library card you can't use the computers." According to Jane, this false assumption of equal access to technology exacerbated the iniquitous experiences of her clients. She bewailed, "People rely too much on everybody having the same access to everything and that's not always the case. They [healthcare providers] need to ask, 'What is the best way to communicate with you? Why aren't you coming in? Why can't we call you? Why can't you call us?'"

Jane's observation highlights how the compounding and reciprocal nature of lack of access to resources negatively impacts her clients' ability to achieve well-being. Additionally, this lack of access to technology complicates the relationship between clients and healthcare professionals, the latter of which sometimes view clients as willfully noncompliant for "failing" to adhere to a treatment plan when, in fact, the client could not and cannot comply because of the lack of access to technology. However, as Jane emphasizes, CHWs can circumvent these issues by advocating that healthcare providers *ask* patients how they should best reach and communicate with them. In terms of assuaging issues of communication, Jane extrapolated that she is sometimes able to find clients low-cost cellphones or other ways to connect clients to the internet. Her example demonstrates how structural factors cause a communication breakdown between patients and medical professionals and how CHWs can remedy such situations by informing medical professionals and through the provision of resources.

As mentioned earlier, some participants described a frustrating issue of learning about a resource that had been present for some time even though they had no prior knowledge of its existence. Carmen, a CHW with more than a decade of experience who works closely with the Latinx immigrant community in south central Indiana, described a case where she was trying to help a Mexican immigrant mother find low-cost eyeglasses for her son. Carmen and the mother had planned to go to a local supermarket in the near future to obtain these eyeglasses. Prior to going to the supermarket, Carmen joined a trip with a group of CHWs and, in passing conversation, learned how she could secure a pair of free eyeglasses within her local community:

> In the van, somebody said, "You know they can get free glasses through the vision 'so-and-so program' at the school district." I'm like, "What?!" I literally got on the phone [with her client] and I was like, "Hold off on that Walmart [to buy glasses]." [I] hooked them up with the school nurse who knew [about] the program. Why they [her client's family] didn't know about it? Probably because something came by in English or the first day with the teacher in school and that didn't come up.

These examples highlight that despite being deeply connected within the local economy and serving as repositories of local, state, and federal resources, CHWs were sometimes quite understandably unaware of resources due to the fluid and ever-changing landscape. These could be present for only a brief amount of time, seemingly disappearing overnight or in a matter of days. Other participants described disparities in resources by county and municipality—even between neighboring counties and cities. This served as an additional stressor and challenge that negatively impacted CHWs and, as a result, their clients who often desperately needed resources. This situation complicated the ability to develop a centralized database of resources and was mentally taxing for the CHW, who had to maintain an ever-changing database in their mind. These challenges were often taken as a personal failure by participants whose moral obligations to their clients and communities were an essential motivator within the moral economy of care. Even when situations like these occurred, CHWs remained resolute and continued their service to clients.

Access to Transportation

Public transportation, or lack thereof, was a predominant social determinant of health described by participants.[29] This served as a major challenge for many clients and communities throughout all parts of Indiana. The lack of public transportation, or of efficient public transportation, caused clients to miss appointments, free services (e.g., health fairs), and job opportunities. Jane explained that even for clients who had access to Medicaid, which would pay for a cab service to take them to appointments, there were still issues. She described that *one trip* to a medical professional appointment used to mean "one round trip"; however, recent changes had made it so that Medicaid covered only one part of the trip—the ride there or the ride home. Other participants noted similar issues related to transportation. Thus, aside from the client being in a tough position, CHWs felt pressured to drive clients to their appointments despite many being, typically, not free to do so for liability reasons. Some CHWs had access to bus passes to distribute to clients, provided by their employers, but many lacked these resources and described feeling pressured to take clients in their personal cars. Relatively few CHWs in this study were covered by liability insurance or used a company care to transport clients. The majority were unable to offer transportation.

Structural and Organizational Barriers

Finally, CHWs described challenges experienced within the organizational infrastructure of their employers. Carmen, who was also employed as a medical interpreter, had, in addition to the work she did in her primary position, also worked with her employer to craft a *promotores de salud* program. Unfortunately, this program was not institutionalized in the hospital where she worked despite the significant need in the local community. Carmen expressed that while her immediate supervisor and she had developed the infrastructure for the program from the ground up, it was frustrating not to have additional support for a needed program such as this. Similarly, Renata, a CHW with 17 years of experience, was hired by a county health department to conduct outreach within the Latinx community. She also had to develop her position from the ground up. Other participants described issues in which organizations would hire a volunteer to serve as a CHW but would lose valuable knowledge if that volunteer CHW left and had not formally structured or developed the position. Carmen lamented that this would result in needing to restart the position from scratch each time. As a result, the structure, or lack thereof, provided by employers could produce negative effects on the ability of CHWs to effectively navigate the moral economy of care.

SUMMARIZING THE MORAL ECONOMY OF CARE

Understanding the structural forces impacting the work of CHWs, such as laws, policies, perceptions of deservingness, and the social determinants of health, is essential to identifying not only the challenges for CHWs and their clients but also the ways in which these workers can be aided to help them become more efficacious. This is especially important for those who have a stake in the successful operation of CHW programs in Indiana, and elsewhere, as these challenges were out of the control of the participants but significantly impacted them as they sought to provide care and resources. Although participants described the need for a centralized database of resources, constructing such a database is difficult given the fluidity of resources and the difficulty in determining whether clients qualify for said resources. Participants described not knowing of resources until too late and/or becoming aware of a resource only after that had existed for some time. These issues create repercussions in the moral economy between CHWs and their clients, keeping CHWs from guiding clients to resources or from doing so in a timely manner.

Structural issues such as nonexistent or inefficient public transportation and lack of access to technology (such as cellphones and internet) were additional barriers that negatively impacted the ability of clients to achieve well-being. Clients were often unable to make appointments (with CHWs or medical professionals), attend free health classes, or travel to job opportunities. The burden would shift to CHWs to provide transportation due to the relationship built between themselves and the client but would unfairly compromise CHWs if they were pressured to provide transport themselves due to liability issues. This balancing act not only placed CHWs in precarious positions, especially if their clients had missed several appointments or needed to establish care, but also hurt their relationships with clients, who could come to see them as unwilling or unable to step up. Similar issues abounded for clients who did not have access to technology such as computers, cellphones, or the internet (a lack of access due, typically, to their not being able to afford it). Some CHWs had access to bus passes (from their employers) or attempted to find deals and free technology (such as securing free or low-cost cellphones or recommending that clients visit the public library to use the internet or securing free or low-cost cellphones), but such work-arounds only went so far.

Policy-makers, employers, and potential employers of CHWs must take into account structural factors, racism and discrimination, and social determinants of health and how these factors shape the moral economy of care. If they do, they will be better able to facilitate the caregiving of these workers. Understanding the impact of these systemic forces will help them to unlock the potential of CHWs. Taking steps like developing policies and descriptions of roles and responsibilities will help employers guarantee the success of CHWs by integrating them into the broader workforce and anticipate and clear barriers to success.

CHWs in Indiana function in ways similar to those described by Nading.[30] In many ways, CHWs act as the disciplining arm of biomedicine, and while CHWs extend the reach of biomedicine from the clinic to the community, they simultaneously act as sources of support and advocates for their clients. In doing so, they fight back against the reductionist approach of biomedicine by illuminating and combating the deleterious impacts of the social determinants of health, thereby facilitating the care provided to their clients. This necessary balancing act highlights how CHWs maintain a tenuous medical citizenship within the moral economy of care as they seek to improve the health and well-being of their clients.[31] Moreover, through witnessing[32] and drawing inspiration from their belief systems (e.g., religions, moral obligations and understandings, and/or compassion), CHWs soften the medical gaze in their caregiving.

The structural factors discussed earlier molded the moral economy of care in which CHWs and their clients operate and enacted boundaries that CHWs either stayed within or crossed in the pursuit of care. At other times, these factors served as barriers that prevented access to care and the ability for CHWs to provide needed resources. I will also show how CHWs exercised agency in helping to reshape the moral economy of care, particularly via their advocacy (detailed in chapter 5). Ultimately, the moral economy of care within which CHWs work is shaped by a variety of overarching structural forces that exert influence and power over micro-level relations. The next chapter examines this moral economy of care further by centering on the CHW-client relationship and the various micro-level factors that shape its reality.

NOTES

1. Fassin 2012: 266.
2. Fassin 2013.
3. Closser 2015; Maes 2012, 2017; Maes et al. 2015a, Nading 2013; Swartz 2013; Swartz and Colvin 2015.
4. Maes 2012.
5. Closser 2015.
6. Maes 2015b, Swartz and Colvin 2015.
7. Swartz and Colvin 2015.
8. Watters 2007.
9. Artiga and Hinton 2018.

10. Indiana ranked as 48 out of 50 states for public health spending with $55 per capita (America's Health Rankings 2020).

11. Mays and Smith 2011.

12. Allen et al. 2014, Kane et al. 2016, Ryabov 2014.

13. Wilkinson and Kleinman 2016: 162.

14. Bovbjerg et al. 2013, Shah et al. 2014.

15. Bovbjerg et al. 2013.

16. Ibid.

17. Maricopa County Department of Public Health 2013.

18. I provide further details on this topic in chapter 2.

19. Also known as "diabetic shock," and occurs when blood sugar levels drop dangerously low.

20. French philosopher Michel Foucault (1994) describes the medical gaze as a dehumanizing medical process that separates the patient's identity from their body, occurring during diagnosis and treatment.

21. Nading 2013.

22. Colvin and Swartz 2015.

23. Davenport 2000.

24. Ibid.

25. Ibid.: 317.

26. Nading 2013.

27. The latter being an issue of concern as distrust of CHWs could spread to others in the community, a topic I discuss in chapter 2.

28. Logan 2020.

29. Ibid.

30. Nading 2013.

31. Ibid.

32. Davenport 2000.

Chapter 2

Connecting with Clients and Engendering Empowerment

Analyzing the CHW-Client Relationship

In September 2017, I visited a large city in southwestern Indiana to meet with a CHW named Andrés, a middle-aged CHW with over a decade of experience who is also trained as a medical interpreter. He originally came to the United States from Latin America and has spent more than 20 years in this town in Indiana. Andrés began his work as a volunteer serving the Latinx immigrant community. He eventually trained as a CHW and began working at a small clinic, making him unique as many CHWs were not employed in this capacity within a biomedical workplace (i.e., employed as a "community health worker"). Though Andrés has responsibilities in the clinic as a medical interpreter, his employer also provides him with a significant amount of dedicated hours to be spent within the community conducting outreach. He also develops health fairs, arranging one as a health outreach program to serve migrant farmworkers who come through the state in the summer months following the harvest.

While shadowing Andrés at the clinic, I waited for him in between his appointments. During his breaks, I asked him about his motivation for being a CHW. He told me, "The community, the people. The love for people. I really love to work for people in need." Andrés told me of his decision to remain in the United States, which proved difficult for him. Nevertheless, he persevered, explaining, "All [of the] different obstacles that I went through after making the decision to stay in the United States by myself, it really allows me to grow more internally, personally, spiritually, mentally, everything because of that experience." For Andrés, drawing on these experiences and the focus on the client is at the core of his motivation for being a CHW. He continued, "Those years of experience having those different obstacles really strengthened my desire to work for the community, even more every day that I work as a community health worker, and I see the different types of problems or needs." Most importantly, for Andrés, drawing on his experience and seeing the needs in the community "completely continues increasing the desire to be a community health worker to help those people in need." Aside from assessing how overarching structural forces impact the moral economy of care as detailed in chapter 1, unpacking the relationships, obligations, motivations, and drives that connect CHWs to their community, employer, and broader society lends further insights into the boundaries that exist within these micro-level relationships.

Other anthropologists have explored how macro-level forces in the form of policy, public health outreach, and other forces shape the moral economy and micro-level relationships between individuals.[1] This approach is particularly useful in examining the relationship that CHWs maintain with their clients and community. As such, moral economy is a prism through which to assess and understand these various realities of CHWs and how they navigate their relationships.

In building relationships with their clients and broader communities, CHWs had to first gain the trust and rapport of their clients. This was further augmented through engagement, outreach, provision of services, and following up with clients to ensure care was received. Participants noted how breakdowns in the relationship could occur if a poor referral was given or if the CHW was unable to speak knowledgeably to the concerns or needs of the client. Other breakdowns in the moral economy of care could occur as news of a failure or fractured relationship could spread throughout the community, thereby damaging the reputation of the CHW.

In describing caregiving in a cancer ward in Botswana, Julie Livingston writes that "care-giving is a moral endeavor. It is at once deeply personal and deeply social, and it is a vital practical matter, crucial to patient well-being and survival."[2] Likewise, CHWs draw on their morals and leverage resources in the moral economy of care when engaging in the practice of caregiving. This chapter builds upon the previous one in taking a closer look at how broader structural forces that shape the moral economy of care impact the relationship between CHWs and their clients. A core feature within the relationship between CHW and the client is building self-sufficiency and engendering empowerment on part of the client. Although CHWs stated their commitment to helping others and always being available, the overarching aim was for clients to become empowered over their health and well-being. Thus, the motivations, qualities, and values held by CHWs intimately shape the moral economy of care and relationships forged between these workers and their clients.

Participants identified a variety of underlying factors that shape their commitment to their clients and how they draw on these in building their relationship such as client motivation, morals, and values possessed by the CHW, and shared demographic characteristics (e.g., race, ethnicity, gender, language, and culture). The ability for CHWs to lead clients to greater self-sufficiency and whether or not this activity was successful had significant impacts that shaped the relationship between these workers and their clients. Participants also experienced a variety of challenges related to these factors and had to find ways to navigate situations in which a client wants to do something outside of their moral compass.

COMPASSION, EMPATHY, AND TRUSTWORTHINESS: ESSENTIAL QUALITIES AND FACTORS IN BECOMING A CHW

In assessing how the moral economy of care affects the relationship between these workers and their clients, participants identified several characteristics that are requisite for CHWs to successfully serve clients and the broader community. The most commonly identified factor was compassion for community and client. This was a critical trait to be possessed by a CHW and was mentioned in over 30 interviews. Participants noted that compassion in addition to trustworthiness and empathy were essential for a CHW to possess and could be trained in the other technical skills of the job. Marcia was one CHW who stressed that compassion was the most essential quality, she asserted, "We can teach you everything else." Martha also echoed Marcia's sentiment and explained, "I don't think passion is something you can really teach. Not just say, 'I want to be a community health worker' to have a job . . . but my personal feeling is you really have to have a passion and deep roots within a community to be able to do that." Compassion combined with a connection to the community and a shared, lived experience comprised the core of being a CHW; without these, there is no CHW. An additional innate quality that participants noted was the ability to be extroverted to navigate the community, to build relationships, to learn the economy of resources, and to advocate for clients and the broader community.

Aside from possessing these innate qualities, many participants described their role of a CHW in a similar regard. When asked how long they had been a CHW, many described a professional timespan and an additional, informal length of time. While a participant may state, for instance, that they have nine years of work experience, they might add that they have additional years of experience in similar capacities. Some even added that their formative years included experiences of helping others as volunteers when they were children. These participants asserted that through their moral obligation to family, friends, and community—in conjunction with their volunteerism—that the essence of being a CHW had been present within them throughout their lifetime.

Other participants had been unaware that there was a specific job title associated with this type of work. Some had served as volunteers or worked in a similar capacity for an organization or clinic as part-time employees. In August 2017, I traveled to southwestern Indiana to meet with Carla, a Latinx woman in her late 20s who worked as a CHW in a small clinic. When I asked Carla how long she had been a CHW, she stated that although she possessed almost three years of experience at her current job, she had worked in a similar capacity or as a volunteer for much longer, exclaiming, "I just never knew what it was called!" Despite her unawareness of the title, she had been driven by her dedication to her community and a strong moral stance toward improving their health outcomes.

The findings presented here connect to the previous work of Bourgois,[3] Horton,[4] and Nading[5] that draw on moral economy to elucidate how the broader politcal economic context affects individuals and how they form social bonds and are driven through motivations, values, and morals. As noted by Martha, in addition to the identified qualities, it is through their connection to the community that cements the relationship and obligation of the CHW and the client.

TRUST, RAPPORT, AND UNDERSTANDING: BUILDING AND MAINTAINING THE CHW-CLIENT RELATIONSHIP

Trust and rapport are central aspects of the relationship between CHWs and their clients. Trust was particularly emphasized as a crucial aspect of the relationship, particularly as a means from which CHWs inspired clients and aided them in achieving well-being. In our conversations, Andrés explained how building trust facilitates openness between the CHW and client, stating, "I will say . . . to be a trustworthy person, you have to also show your concern, your credibility, be sincere with the person, not just because you're being paid but it's a combination—you have to be putting yourself in front of them, open to them, in order for them to be open to you." He further emphasized that you must "establish that rapport" and continually build the relationship. Through trust, the CHW demonstrates their credibility and sincerity within the moral economy of care and, according to Andrés, this supersedes the fact that CHWs are compensated for their labor.

Other participants noted that gaining trust was often the first challenge to overcome when establishing care with a new client. Dean, a White CHW in his mid-60s, explained that earning clients' trust and establishing it as central within the relationship was challenging. He stated "[It's challenging] trying to get the people to trust you. Because without the trust you don't have anything. Everything else is just the details. You have to have the trust." Earning and building upon trust in the CHW-client relationship was essential in providing care and, without this, the CHW will be unable to bring their client toward empowerment.

In the pursuit of building trust and rapport with clients, the unpaid labor of CHWs is highlighted. Some participants described their attempts to foster relationships with clients after the workday had ended. These participants explained they would not turn off their work cellphone after ending the day just in case a client called who was in need. Andrés told me that he gave his clients his personal cellphone number—a practice forbidden by his employer—so that clients could always reach him. While this provided round-the-clock service that reinforced their relationship, Andrés risked experiencing burnout as a result of always being available (a topic that I cover in-depth in chapter 6). Others described helping clients or individuals in public or serving as a volunteer in their spare time. These extra steps taken by CHWs were done in the pursuit of fostering connections and demonstrating their commitment to clients and community. This connection to the community was cited by participants as central to aiding clients and situated at the heart of the moral economy of care. From this basis, CHWs could begin to provide services and resources, with the goal of building empowerment and self-sufficiency for clients and community.

As described in chapter 1, there was the potential for pitfalls that could damage the CHW-client relationship. Participants noted this particularly when connecting clients with resources and making referrals to medical professionals and social service organizations. While successful referrals reinforced the bond between CHW and their client, referrals that did not result in the needed services or resources could damage this relationship, possibly jeopardizing it entirely. When I asked Beverly about how referrals and resource provision affected the relationship between CHWs and clients, she stated,

> You need to be [aware of resources] because I know for a fact that if you're not on top of things and you're dealing with the community and you start telling people things that are not quite true, believe me when you're out in the public they'll [clients/community] be saying, "Don't deal with her [the CHW] because she doesn't really know her job." And that's not what a community health worker wants to hear.

In order to address this issue, participants stressed that follow-up was an essential practice after making a referral. Follow-up occurred most often in the form of a call or visit with the clients and served as a mechanism to ensure that clients accessed the resources that the resources served their intended purpose, and/or appropriate treatment was provided at medical or social services appointments. Positive referrals strengthened the relationship, while a negative referral *could* damage it. If there had been a negative interaction, participants asserted it was the responsibility of the CHW to rectify this issue and connect clients to other resources or services. Through this action, a negative referral could be corrected and not risk damage to the relationship.

Overall, the qualities identified that make an ideal CHW combined with fostering trust with clients are interwoven within their approach to care. In developing this trust, CHWs could push clients to supersede boundaries and barriers that prevented their ability to attain well-being. Care in the case of the CHW is expanded to encompass not only biomedical health care but also social well-being. While at the surface much of the work performed by CHWs appears to be strictly health related, they also take into account the constellation of social needs of their clients in the pursuit of achieving total well-being.

BUILDING SELF-SUFFICIENCY AND ENGENDERING EMPOWERMENT

Once CHWs had established a relationship and developed rapport with clients, they would set out on the path of identifying barriers, needs, and finding ways to empower clients to take ownership of their health and well-being. CHWs would then work to provide the necessary services and resources to help clients in their path toward health. This relationship built on improving health and well-being was not one of the interminable handholding. CHWs expected their clients to learn how to overcome barriers preventing their ability to achieve health, identify resources, and hone their self-sufficiency. This concept was described as *empowerment*, in which the CHW served as the primary actor who would engender this outcome. Within the moral economy of care, the relationship between the CHW is essentially a process that via health education, advocacy, provision of resources, and clients' incrementally taking steps toward self-sufficiency that the cycle is completed (i.e., from reliance on CHW to self-sufficiency). This cycle comprises the CHW drawing on their morals, values, obligation, and investing their time and energy to engender empowerment (which, as described in chapter 1, can be mitigated by the broader political context in Indiana).

At the outset, this relationship predominantly consists of client reliance on the worker. This was to be expected as the CHW provided health education, resources, and served as an advocate in order to provide the necessary assistance to the client. As the CHW continued to provide assistance, there was an expectation that the client would begin to take steps in his or her own health and life decisions. This could also include things such as maintaining a regular exercise routine, navigating their environment (e.g., using public transportation, making doctor's appointments, identifying and accessing available resources), asking questions and standing up for oneself to medical professionals, and/or integrating proper nutrition into their dietary needs. Participants were quick to note that they would always be there for the client to rely on but that working toward self-sufficiency was the ultimate goal. Bianca, a CHW, summarized this by stating, "The most important part of being a community health worker is empowering the client; showing worth and dignity to the client and equipping them to improve their whole health."

Empowerment was engendered by CHWs through a variety of activities and actions. Participants described calling to schedule appointments at various medical and nonmedical places for clients, such as doctor's offices, insurance companies, and/or social service organizations. Usually, the CHW would place a three-way call that also included the client. In the following calls, the CHW would take a less forward role in the call thereby giving more agency to the client to schedule the appointment. Participants would continue to coach their client until they would make the call themselves. Rhonda, a CHW, explained how she would initiate the call to the clinic or agency, introduce herself and her role as a CHW, and then allow the client to take over the conversation to allow them to develop communication skills and engender empowerment. The engendering of empowerment was essential within the moral economy of care between CHW and client. While these workers placed the needs of their client and community at the forefront, they expected to see clients become empowered as a sign of success following the provision of aid, education, and any other resources.

This was also seen in how these workers described not simply giving away tools and resources to overcome social determinants of health, but through clients exercise their own agency in using these tools and resources. While I spent time shadowing Andrés, he spoke about the importance of not just providing resources but "guiding them to help themselves." The tools, education, and resources are one step in this process that leads to empowerment. Many of the participants took a similar stance in that they wanted to see their clients lead healthier and more fulfilling lives but with the caveat that they are able to utilize these tools on their own accord.

Isabella described how sometimes engendering empowerment within clients is by simply helping them to realize that the solution to their seemingly large problem is a small step forward. To help her clients come to this realization, she takes on the role of an informal counselor, listens to her client's issues, and helps them to reassess the problem from a different angle. She captured a visual representation of this process during the photovoice project in answering the prompt: "What is an impact you have had as a CHW? (see figure 2.1)"

Isabella explicated that she realized in her work as a CHW, she helps clients discern a clearer vision for themselves and how to navigate the barriers presented by various issues in their lives as one means to engender empowerment. "I feel like this picture as you walk closer to the water, you are able to see the clear skies, you are able to see and breathe pure air," Isabella stated. She continued, "Personally, I feel that and I know that our clients feel the same way when that blindfold is removed and I feel very blessed to have the honor and the opportunity to help them sometimes see a little clearer."

In order to engender empowerment within the moral economy of care, CHWs had to be cognizant of a myriad of resources, know how to access and deliver them, understand barriers in the community, and draw on their moral obligation to their clients. Following the development of a trusting relationship and building rapport with clients, CHWs could begin their provision of services and resources in return for seeing clients becoming empowered and increasingly self-sufficient.

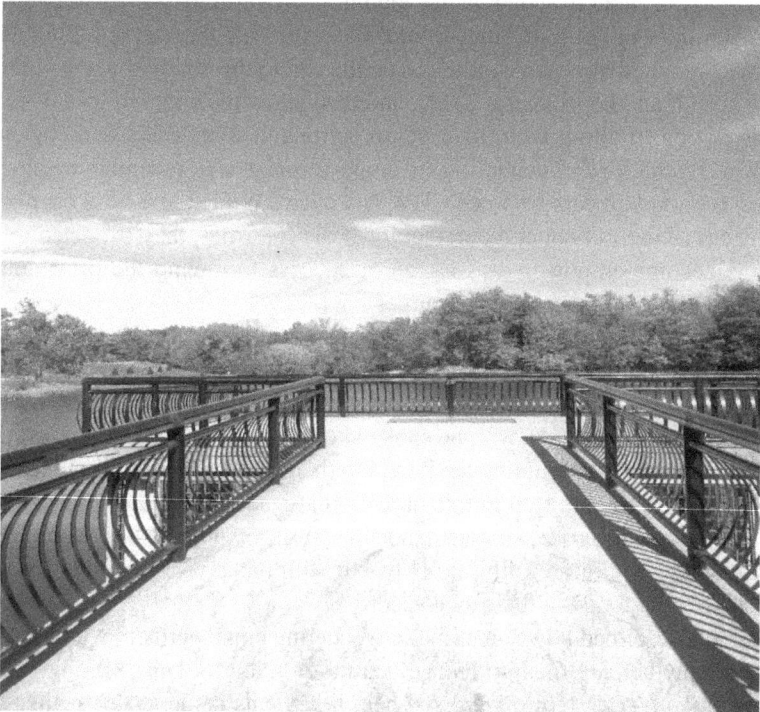

Figure 2.1 **"A clearer picture can be seen when the blindfolds have been removed."**
Source: Photo by Isabella (Pseudonym).

A Critique and a Response to Engendering Empowerment

Much as it can be argued that CHWs extend the dehumanizing and reduction-ist medical gaze within their communities, a similar argument can be made of engendering empowerment. One that CHWs extend the neoliberal approach toward health and well-being, which underscores that the individual is solely responsible for their own health and health behaviors. As such, it can be argued that CHWs are simply reproducing this approach toward health and well-being with their clients and within their communities. However, I argue—in the same vein in chapter 1 regarding the medical gaze—that CHWs mitigate this neolib-eral approach and responsibilization of health. While it is true that participants sought to help clients to take control over their health and well-being, they were always there as a resource and guide for clients. CHWs also did not stop their work at engendering empowerment either. Participants also demonstrated their dedication to clients via advocacy as a form of caregiving in addressing the social determinants of health that deleteriously affect their communities. In this way, changing the landscape by reducing the impacts of structural vulner-ability and improving the health choices of their communities. Although CHWs may extend the reach of the neoliberal approach, they actively subverted and upended this approach and political economic environment which places their clients and communities at a disadvantage.

This approach taken by CHWs is similar to that taken by Latinx nurses who provided care to undocumented migrants despite these patients being consid-ered undeserving of care.[6] While operationalizing the neoliberal approach of self-sufficiency and responsibility, Latinx nurses "hybridized" neoliberal values and social justice (e.g., health as a human right, compassion for com-munity) to provide care. Lo and Nguyen argue, "Latinx nurses resisted the racialization of medical un-deservingness against co-ethnic immigrants."[7] In demonstrating how their patients were "becoming" self-sufficient, they underscored their medical deservingness. In addition to Lo and Nguyen,[8] other scholars have also documented how healthcare workers and advocacy groups mix this neoliberalism approach to health with social justice values in the pursuit of care.[9] Similarly, CHWs in this project drew on shared ethnicity as well as race and other sociodemographic factors in connecting with clients and providing care.

RACE AND ETHNICITY IN THE CHW-CLIENT RELATIONSHIP AND ENGENDERING EMPOWERMENT

Sharing sociodemographic factors with clients, including race, ethnicity, culture, language, gender, class, and education, were powerful connectors in the CHW-client relationship. When I inquired about the impact of sharing the same racial or ethnic background, Beverly stated, "Because you're part of the community, you know the needs of the community. Another part is you look like them. You . . . know their struggles . . . and they know that you are not just there to sugar coat anything." She asserted, "I found that in my years of training that people tend to want to be empowered to do things when they know and they see people that look like them." While sharing the same racial or ethnic background between CHW and client is not a prerequisite for being a CHW, many participants also expressed that possessing these shared sociodemographic factors did indeed help to foster the relationship and could be leveraged to empower clients.

It should also be noted that participants stressed they would never discriminate or only serve clients of the same racial and/or ethnic background. Rather, CHWs could leverage these shared factors to engender empowerment within clients by demonstrating how they had overcome their shared structural vulnerability and thereby serve as a role model for their clients. These workers also leveraged other sociodemographic characteristics such as level of education and social class as additional factors to engender empowerment.

Having a shared ethnic or cultural background was especially important for Latinx immigrants and Spanish-speaking clients served by CHWs. Magdalena, a volunteer CHW and an English as a second language teaching assistant, told me, "I try to help people because at one point I was like them when I came to the U.S. twenty-three years ago and I got the help I needed. I'm thankful. I have been in their shoes." Interacting with a CHW who shares an immigrant experience in addition to language served as a means to connect with clients. These factors quickly established a relationship between the CHW and client and were useful in communicating with clients to overcome health and social issues they experienced as a result of structural violence.

However, sharing the same racial or ethnic background does not always signify that an immediate connection can be made and can be hindered by a lack of shared, lived experience or level of education. Beverly told me about one of her friends, who is a medical doctor and person of color and how the white coat worn by medical professionals can yield negative impacts in their interaction with the community. She stated, "When they [medical professionals] wear their white coat . . . and they go into a poor community, the community sometimes shuts down, because they figure that you think you're higher than them—even though you look like them," Beverly explained, "I think we [CHWs] have an understanding, not that that person doesn't have an understanding because they do, but it's their mindset. They [the clients] feel intimidated just by that coat." This concept of the "white coat syndrome"[10] was echoed by other participants, explaining that their clients would feel excluded or powerless in the interaction with the medical professional. Beverly elaborated how it was possible for barriers to be enacted between medical professionals in a race/ethnic concordant relationship with a patient, stating,

> I know for a fact that when you have laypeople that are dealing with professionals, even though they could be the same race, there's a disconnect there because they [the laypeople] think that your word is gospel, [that] the professional word is gospel. And what they're really feeling about themselves and their health [is] that the doctor knows best and they don't. But when you have a doctor that gives you that arrogance—that can be a negative effect because that client is not going to open up to you. They're not gonna advocate for themselves because you [the medical professional] have the degree. "What do you know [about your own health]?" And that does happen a lot . . . you have the "professional ethnicity." It could happen a lot because of that superiority if you will.

Beverly's example highlights the limits of sharing race or ethnicity between a patient and a medical professional due to the "professional ethnicity" of the latter. CHWs, on the other hand, circumvent this power dynamic through not only connecting with clients on a racial and ethnic level but through other factors such as similar education, shared lived experience, and social class. I asked other participants to elaborate on the dynamics of being in a race and/or ethnic concordant relationship with clients. Alisha described how shared race is a pivotal factor in the provision of health care. She echoed Beverly's prior example and explained, "What does it look like having a Black family or ...whatever, and all you see is the white coats or White people, White people, White people all the time? Like I want to be able to relate to somebody else who really understands me, who *really* understands *me*."

Alisha's example was further highlighted by Beverly, who critiqued outsiders who come into the community in order to "help" and who also do not share a similar racial and/or ethnic background:

> You get someone who wants to come in [to our organization] and give you classes—and they've never been in the trenches! "So, you wrote a [health] program?" You've never even been to the trenches. How are you going to sit there and try to help someone and you've never been where they are? You never have to deal trying to figure out how your child is going to get milk or how to keep the heat on. You have no clue why they can't go to the doctor—because they have no transportation! Honestly, you can't be White and come and tell me how to do things. You haven't been in my shoes. Of course people aren't going to listen to you!

In her example, race discordance and the lack of shared lived experience combine to cause breakdowns in the provision of care, resources, and health

education. However, between CHWs and clients, Beverly added how sharing lived experience and the same racial background can foster successful
relationships:

> It's really a positive factor. Because . . . they're people that look like you. And
> because I run into this all the time, people open up better when it's somebody
> of their own race. Because they think they figured that you understand a lot of
> the things that they're going through or you've heard about it and then it's not
> foreign to you. So, yeah, I think they have a better understanding.

These examples from Beverly and Alisha highlight how outsiders, especially those not of the same racial or ethnic background as the community,
can fail when attempting to provide care or implement health programs. This
also underscores the need for health programs to be collaborative in scope
with CHWs and the community members in order to be successful. This is
vital given that CHWs experienced or continue to be affected by the same
structural vulnerabilities as their clients and can draw upon these experiences in order to foster deep connections with clients to facilitate health and
well-being and, thereby, ensure the success of such outreach by outsiders.
Similarly, other CHWs may leverage their own experiences with substance
use disorder, mental health disorders, and/or incarceration in order to build
relationships with clients.

Other CHWs, such as Martha and Carmen, spoke to the ability to speak
the same language as superseding shared race or ethnicity. Carmen stated,
"It makes a difference even if the doctor is not from their ethnic background
but speaks the language. It makes a difference because once they are hearing their own language, they are more up to asking more questions or if
they have a doubt or to feel more comfortable." Previous research has also
demonstrated positive correlations between speaking the same language,
which can provoke positive interactions regardless of race and ethnic
concordance.[11]

Participants strongly expressed being able to serve and advocate for clients
and communities outside of their racial and ethnic backgrounds. Carmen
explained how, despite some potential initial hesitation, deep connections can
be fostered quickly "but when they see that you really care, Black folks [and]
some White folks telling us all about how unhealthy their lives are and we're
like, 'Oh, what is this White person talking about?'—15 minutes later—'Girl!
That's what just happened to me!' And once you're in [accepted], they will go
out in the street and kill for you. Once you get past that little thing." However,
Carmen acknowledged that ideally the CHW should come from within the
said community, "But ideally I would say yes, from your own community is
better." Overall, sharing the same racial and/or ethnic background was seen

by participants as a positive factor in establishing relationships with clients and improving well-being.

Analyzing Race and Ethnic Concordance in the CHW-Client Relationship

Despite participants' assertions that racial and ethnic concordance produced positive connections and outcomes with clients, there is evidence that contradicts that concordance is a positive factor in building relationships, especially in healthcare interactions in which there exists heightened power dynamics. Several studies have demonstrated that racial concordance between physician and patient produces little to no positive outcomes or can actually cause a negative effect within the relationship.

Blanchard et al.[12] found racial concordance between physician and patient to not always serve as a positive factor. In this study, Latinx patients were more likely to report "being treated with disrespect" if their physician had the same racial or ethnic background. However, their study also showed that these feelings were stratified between racial groups—with Asian and White respondents less likely to report being treated unfairly if they were racially concordant with their provider. Overall, Blanchard et al.[13] argue that other factors such as cultural and sociodemographic factors must be accounted for in assessing the provider-patient relationship.

Other studies have shown little impact when it comes to race and ethnic concordance in the physician-patient relationship. Kumar et al.[14] assessed the perceived quality of care by Black and White patients and found that race concordance had no bearing on the perceived quality of care. They also controlled for income, sex, age, insurance status, type of insurance, and education and still found no impacts. Kumar et al.[15] found that for White patients, only education income and insurance status were associated with perceived quality of care, whereas Black patients associated higher satisfaction of perceived quality of care with education.

Several studies have demonstrated how shared language and communication skills—especially for Latinx and Black patients—have produced positive health outcomes. Traylor et al.[16] revealed positive health outcomes for Spanish-speaking Latinx patients in adhering to cardiovascular disease medication. Adams et al.[17] conducted a study on the disclosure of depression between physician and Afro-Caribbean patients and found that communication style was more significant compared to race concordance. Their study demonstrated that physicians who had a "high patient-centered" communication style yielded better patient experiences overall. A study conducted by Schoenthaler et al.[18] revealed that communication style and a collaborative relationship between physician and patient in a race discordant relationship produced positive health outcomes compared to less positive health outcomes in a less collaborative relationship. Their study also revealed that race concordance did not produce significant health outcomes.

Diversity within the ancillary medical team (e.g., nurses, receptionists, medical assistants, and, potentially, CHWs) could be a mitigating factor according to Blanchard et al.[19] Similarly, Meghani et al.[20] describe in their review of the literature that the majority of studies that assessed race concordance between physician-patient and not with other staff members. Thus, limiting our understanding of the impacts of race and ethnic concordance with other members of the medical team in the full medical experience. While the participants in this study asserted the positive effects of having a shared background with clients, it should be noted that race, ethnicity, and other sociodemographic factors also impact the provider-client experience.

Recent studies have demonstrated that race and ethnic concordance between CHWs and clients has produced positive health outcomes.[21] Wells et al.[22] revealed that CHWs that share the same race and/or ethnicity as their clients resulted in higher rates of mammography screenings. Similarly, Murayama et al.[23] demonstrated positive results between CHWs in race/ethnic concordant relationships with clients that resulted in greater patient efficacy of diabetes management. Other research has demonstrated positive outcomes between the role of ancillary staff and race concordance.[24] The latter assessed the navigator-patient race and language concordance in cancer screening and demonstrated that race and language concordance were significant factors in improving rates of cancer screening.

Other factors for participants in this study could be that they primarily existed outside the realm of the healthcare team and also shared other factors such as cultural, language, gender, educational, and socioeconomic concordance that facilitated the connection between CHW and client. Indeed, other studies that have explored race and ethnicity assert that other factors are at play in this relationship. Sanders et al.[25] reveal that "personal" and "ethnic" were two categories that were associated with higher satisfaction related to patient navigation and cancer care. They assert that interpersonal characteristics are also important factors aside from race and ethnicity and argue that communication is essential to developing higher levels of trust between physician and patient. Ultimately, social connection is a key factor in developing these relationships. Thus, race and ethnic concordance, a reduced power dynamic, and other factors from the findings presented in this book and previous research highlight a myriad of characteristics CHWs can draw on in developing relationships with clients and producing positive health behaviors and outcomes.

THE ISSUE OF GENDER IN THE
CHW-CLIENT RELATIONSHIP

To a lesser extent, participants also described the positive and negative effects of gender and its impact within the moral economy of care. The majority of CHWs in this sample identified as female (n = 39, ~80 percent) compared to male (n = 10, ~20 percent). Several participants described that being the same gender of their client can help facilitate the establishment of a trusting relationship. Alejandra, a Latinx woman and CHW, told me

> "*También*, it [being the same gender] helps too, between women it makes it easier and easier to trust . . . it's more closed with a man, with women they tell you more. You learn a lot more when it's a woman."

Other participants, such as Martha, explained that training more men as CHWs could serve as another way to connect to male populations. Noting that men might connect more with men, Martha stated, "And that's good [having the two men trained] because there are some clients that do better with someone like them, you know, 'I don't want a lady' or whatever because they may have things, they don't want to privy up on." Thus, being the same gender functioned in a way similar to race and ethnicity in providing an avenue for CHWs to connect with clients.

Carmen recounted to me the issues that arose due to gender in helping middle-aged Latinx male clients at doctor's appointments regarding their sexual health. She explained that she draws on her training as a scientist and tries "to be friendly without being dry." Carmen described a situation in which she was serving in the capacity of a medical interpreter. She had to translate for male patients who were experiencing erectile dysfunction, prostate issues, and to ascertain if particular medicines would produce side effects that could impact their sex life. She told me how she would explain to her client about Health Insurance Portability and Accountability Act (HIPAA) and that information discussed in the appointment is completely confidential. However, she noted how these interactions may be different if she were a younger woman. Carmen described that even for her oldest male client, she is usually at least ten years older than him and thus is not likely to be thought of as a sexual partner, which she described as the "grandma effect." Thus, Carmen's "grandma effect" demonstrates how age plays a mitigating factor in providing health services to clients of different genders.

Isabella explained how it can be initially challenging when helping Latinx male clients. Isabella explained that she draws on her training as a CHW to develop a relationship and to demonstrate that she truly cares about their health. She explained, "I have several males that I serve here and I do feel a little bit of resistance, in the beginning a lot of resistance, but now after building more rapport with them and making sure that they were ok, they started to see that, 'Ok, yeah, she cares, I'll let her in.' And now they feel more comfortable talking to me about how they are feeling and their symptoms and needs are."

However, Isabella explained that she had encountered uncomfortable situations with male clients. She told me, "I guess at times . . . it can be uncomfortable if I'm serving a male, but I have to set it aside and not see them as a gender but as a human that needs help. If I start feeling that sometimes men . . . they give you that stare or wrong hug that makes you feel dirty and it's like, 'Ok, alright, how do I serve this person?'" Isabella expressed developing strategies to overcome these situations, explaining, "I've learned to have tunnel vision and not see that, if they want to be dirty or perverted 'Ok,' but I'm not going to allow that from not giving them the best attention they need. I think it'd be nice [to have more male CHWs] but sometimes the males they don't like to help each other because they feel weird because they don't like discussing the personal private things." Thus, for Isabella, she focuses instead of gender on helping the individual as a fellow human being as much as she can. She also notes that while more male CHWs would potentially be beneficial, it may not overcome male gender stereotypes about not wanting to share health concerns, participate in care work, and other personal topics.

Dean, a male CHW in his 60s, primarily works with an elderly client base. In my conversations with Dean, he told me that his religion serves as a boundary from becoming too involved in helping female clients. Activities such as going into their apartments and talking with them one-on-one are prohibited due to his religiosity. This example stands in contrast to that of other studies, which have noted how religiosity can help overcome such issues of gendered care.[26] Nonetheless, even with elderly male clients, Dean explained that he encounters barriers sometimes stating that they don't reach out for help too much and that if he tries too persistently, they tend to withdraw. Dean called this the "John Wayne syndrome" and explained that his male clients will sometimes even refuse transportation (which, in Dean's case he is able to provide due to his employer providing liability insurance) and would rather pay for a taxi or seek other modes of transportation—as a means to seek care on their own volition without assistance from a CHW.

This disparity in gender of CHWs is unsurprising and found throughout the scholarly work on the topic of CHWs and is reflective of trends in the United States and other countries.[27] In exploring this disparity, Villa-Torres et al.[28] surveyed Latinx men in North Carolina to ascertain their view toward CHW work in addition to the potential health impacts CHW training could produce on men's health. Their study found that Latinx men were often unwilling to participate in CHW programs due to conceptions of "traditional" gender norms, immigration status, and being unable to engage in this type of work, which often went unpaid. Their study highlights the need to understand how gender facilitates or prohibits participation in the utilization of CHW services (and training to become a CHW). Participants in this study, however, described as they did with race and ethnicity that they would help someone of any gender as much as possible—barring some caveats.

These examples demonstrate how gender can be a positive factor or a source of contention in the CHW-client relationship in Indiana. At times, some participants felt serving clients of a different gender was inappropriate depending on client behavior, social context, and/or religious views. Participants drew on other factors in their life, such as age, in order to address issues that arose through helping a client of a different gender. If the issue of gender was too much to overcome, CHWs referred the client to another CHW in order to establish care. Aside from issues in race, ethnicity, and gender, morals and values were additional factors CHWs navigated within the moral economy of care.

MORAL DIVISION IN THE
CHW-CLIENT RELATIONSHIP

Although motivated by a strong moral connection to their communities and clients, participants were, at times, challenged by specific situations depending on the needs and desires of the client. These situations impacted their ability to provide care and resources to clients. Several examples of issues that challenged the morals and values and manifested as potential barriers for participants included abortion, drug use, issues in interpersonal relationships of clients (e.g., intimate partner violence), LBGTQ+ issues, and the use of contraception. In spite of being challenged by these issues, participants emphasized that the health of the client supersedes their religious and moral convictions. The client should be informed, counseled, and provided with appropriate referrals but their autonomy should be at the forefront. If CHWs felt they were unable to reconcile the needs and wishes of the client with their moral standpoint, then the client should be referred to another CHW or service provider who could better assist them with the desired resources and/or services.

Participants described a variety of strategies and responses when they encountered a client whose actions or desires challenged their moral or religious views. CHWs would still try to provide the client with positive and healthy options that would also respect their autonomy while at the same time not compromising their morals and values. This could be a tricky balancing act and at times challenge the CHW's dual medical citizenship.[29] Carmen told me her approach is one that "tr[ies] to focus on what needs [she] can meet for that person without trying to run their life." Andrés expressed a similar view, "First of all, my approach is just to let them know that I'm trying to understand the way they do things but I also let them know my limitations in what I do and what kind of morals and values and principles I have and that I'm also trying to be respectful and trying to focus on the problem in the situation."

Participants still placed the client first in these situations, ensuring that their client is respected that they understand their clients' needs, but that also recognized their own limitations. Camila, a Latinx CHW in her early 30s who works for a women's clinic in a large hospital in Indianapolis, told me that in helping her female clients to make choices about their sexual health and pregnancy, she ultimately tells her clients that they are the ones who must make the final choice about their health. Camila told me, "It's not my scope of practice to try to change anything in them," elaborating, "but to say, 'Hey, you have a future, study for your future, want more out of your future. You probably don't want kids now but [maybe] in the future—because you will be more prepared to take care of your kids . . . It's ok, you have many options here [in the U.S.].'" Her approach demonstrates that she does not want to necessarily "change anything" in terms of the client's decisions but rather to empower them to see a different future and let the client determine the best option.

Gabriela, a Latinx woman and a CHW, recounted a similar approach in which she does not try to force change upon a client but rather tries to get them to see how a decision might reverberate into their future. When I asked her if she had ever been in a situation in which a client wanted to do something that went against her morals, she stated,

> Hmm . . . I had that with a person that wanted to seek out an abortion. I mean that definitely goes against my personal morals but I just really try to help them understand not only what their choice is for the moment but I ask the clients can you live with this choice six months, six years away? Are you going to be able to handle what you made a decision on? So, I would say that's probably the biggest [perspective]: can you live with it? See a longer span. I find that a lot of people in crisis or in poverty have a short-range view. Their view is immediate because they are in crisis . . . so I think part of my job is to expand that horizon so I say, "Ok, let's look at it from a different angle."

For other participants, their religious conviction strongly influenced their foundation from which they help clients but also for when they had to remove themselves from actions taken by clients that challenged this foundation.

Beverly noted how her religion was vital to her work and served as a guiding compass that she could not sway on:

> We don't do that [something against the morals/values]. If it's against my morals, I will let them know. I haven't ran across that gap, but I have to answer to God. I don't do something that is against His will. I will explain to you [the client] why I won't. . . . And I'm not going to disrespect what you want to do but if it's against my personal morals, I won't do it. I will give you a reason but I'm not going to discuss how you see it because it's not going to sway me. Because if I sway on that, I'll sway on anything.

Beverly notes how if she were flexible in terms of her moral guidelines, she may sway on other issues. She demonstrates that she ultimately respects the will of the client but will remove herself from the situation if need be. Dean expressed a similar viewpoint, "I would tell them that I want to help you, but I have a certain belief that prevents me from doing it this time but I can and will arrange for you to meet with another person that might be of your same beliefs that would not present a problem." In another example, Bob, a cross-trained paramedic and CHW, described how he approached helping a client who wanted to do something that went against his morals. He described a conversation he had trying to persuade a client to go to the emergency room. Bob told me, "I've had that on the ambulance before [something that challenged his moral standpoint]," recounting an interaction with a client:

[Client]: No, I don't want to go to the hospital.
[Bob]: You are going to die, you are *literally* going to die if you don't go.
[Client]: I don't care.

Bob elaborated, "You know, you can't kidnap them, if they're of sound mind and they want to stay there and die, you just can't kidnap them. Now, does that morally go against my feelings—hell yes!" He added, "I may not agree with it [the option they are considering], but at least I can try to let them know: here is the healthiest way or safest to go about it, at least try to go through a physician."

Maintaining client agency and respecting the wishes of the client were emphasized during the certification course. The training emphasized that CHWs must be respectful of clients and be sensitive to race, ethnicity, gender, and sexual orientation. While many participants expressed their religion as a key source of inspiration and motivation, they were keenly aware of LGBTQ+ issues and were open to topics such as contraception. Participants were also trained that if they felt they could not effectively aid a client based on a moral conflict, then the client should be transferred to another CHW and/or health/ social service professional who could provide additional information and/or appropriate services. Thus, CHWs were trained in how to navigate difficult relationships while holding the autonomy of the client at the forefront.

CHALLENGES IN THE CHW-CLIENT RELATIONSHIP

Although CHWs were compassionate and sought every way possible to aid their clients, many participants recounted the challenges they faced when engendering empowerment. These challenges ranged from broad structural challenges to idiosyncratic issues. However, when challenges arose, the majority of the participants did not blame clients but rather themselves. Participants often pondered what they were doing wrong and sought new ways of approach to reach out to the client to surmount whatever barrier existed to achieve their well-being.

In spite of providing health fairs and free classes (e.g., information and classes about nutrition, exercise, chronic disease management), garnering community attendance could prove difficult. Several participants lamented that this could be due to a lack of interest within the community. In order to address this, Marcia and her organization changed the format of the classes such as having a 4-hour class instead of an 8-hour class. They also tried to incentivize participation by providing a $10 gift card that could be used for gas or groceries. Other participants described how they would have a class or health fair and provide a free service, such as a mammogram, as an incentive to attend.

Aside from potential structural barriers that prevented attendance at various events, some participants argued that idiosyncratic issues on part of the client served as a barrier to attendance. Rosa, a CHW with 1 year experience but over 20 years as a doula, explained, "Sometimes when they are faced with a challenge because of their health, they create their own barriers . . . [they] isolate themselves." She noted that this is particularly challenging to overcome but that she continually tries to help clients overcome this barrier and take advantage of free services and events in the community. However, some participants noted that it seemed apparent that some clients do not want to become empowered. This was demonstrated by clients who would rather have the CHW continue to make appointments and provide services and resources with no inclination of taking the initiative themselves.

While shadowing Isabella, she recounted a situation that she had been experiencing with one of her clients. This individual seemed to continually rely on her even though she had worked with this individual for some time and had provided them with resources, information, and coaching on the skills necessary to engender empowerment. In this specific case, the client would continually ask her to schedule their prescription refills. And while she continued to help this individual, Isabella began to feel frustrated and hopeless since she had been willing to do everything she could possibly think of but still had been unable to engender empowerment within this individual. And, although it seemed Isabella had done all she could to engender empowerment in this individual, she still sought new ways to lead her client to greater self-sufficiency.

Other participants described that clients did not seem to value the free or subsidized resources offered by the CHW or their organization. Camila described how some of her clients were unsure of utilizing free services offered at the clinic. These clients seemed to question the intrinsic value of this free service when it is offered on a free or sliding fee scale. The assumption on the part of the client, Camila asserted, is that the service must not be "very good" or "effective" since it is being offered at such a reduced value. Camila posed a photograph to encapsulate this challenge, note the use of lower bills (or "free") next to CHW services and the use of higher bills along with cards that symbolize policy, paperwork, and other barriers to attaining the services on the other side (see figure 2.2). She summed up this issue in her caption, in which she states a challenge is "being valued by our clients."

This issue served as a prominent challenge in her outreach and attempts to provide care for her clients and community. Her example underscores a unique challenge in the moral economy. The clients' devalued services that were subsidized or offered for free, connecting the lack of cost to an erroneous notion that the services must also be "cheap" or "not as good." In Camila's

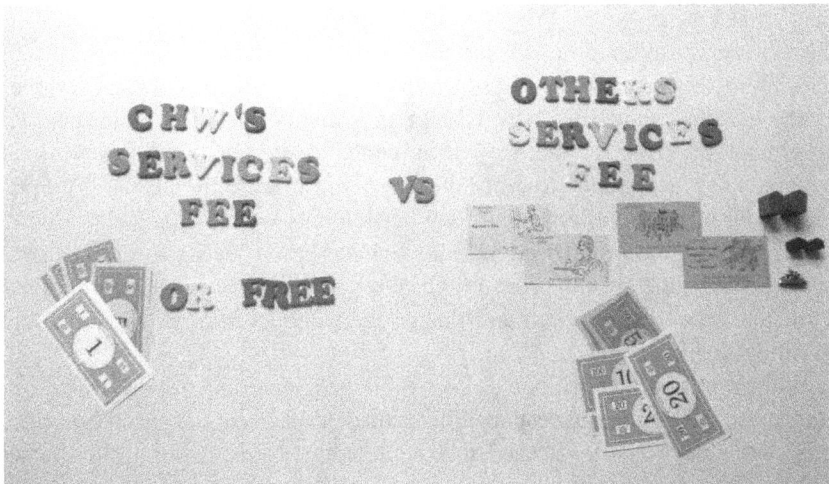

Figure 2.2 **"One of our challenges is being valued by our clients because sometimes we provide our services for free."** *Source:* Photo by Camila (Pseudonym).

perspective, this attitude thereby demonstrated that clients also devalued the overarching CHW-client relationship. Camila asserted that overcoming this mindset was essential in order to provide these services within the community.

Participants described feelings of frustration but also noted the need to manage these emotions so that they do not negatively impact their work. After encountering similar issues and frustration, Andrés described how he must control these negative emotions, stating "sometimes some people can be a little frustrating when you're trying to do something to better their lives and they don't follow up. But it's part of the job that you have to manage your feelings and try to continue to be effective as a CHW." Maricela also managed these emotions, asserting that normally there is a "good reason" why a client does not want to become empowered or does not seem to "have the time." Maricela instead stressed listening and understanding in these instances, saying, "We don't know their stories or their whole stories. So, learning how to listen is the main part of giving and getting good services."

Overall, despite encountering challenges, whether due to structural barriers or idiosyncratic issues, CHWs continued to search for new methods to engender empowerment. These workers always sought to place clients at the forefront via incentivizing participation, managing frustrations, and listening. For many participants, they redirected their frustration to persevere and improve client and community well-being.

MOTIVATING FOR CHANGE: THE MORAL ECONOMY OF CARE AND THE CHW-CLIENT RELATIONSHIP

Ultimately, these relationships are the conduit in which participants infused their morals, values, skills, and services in order to provide care and services to the client. Elucidating how CHWs and clients construct their relationships and analyzing the factors that influence them is essential to reveal the nuances that affect and structure the provision of care by CHWs. The primary goal of this relationship among participants was to engender empowerment. While the broader environment shaped their ability to provide care and services, the moral drive of CHWs provided motivation to address challenges they experienced and that of their clients in order to ameliorate health issues.

While an important critique to levy is how engendering empowerment can reproduce the neoliberal responsibilization within clients affected by structural violence, CHWs softened this approach via empowering clients and emphasizing their deservingness to care.[30] CHWs also nuance this extension of the neoliberal approach in continuing to advocate for clients and circumventing the structural factors affecting their communities (a topic that will be covered further in chapter 5). Within the moral economy of care, CHWs drew on a variety of sociodemographic factors to empower clients and leveraged these to create connections and foster relationships with clients. And while morals were pivotal reasons for participating in this role, when clients sometimes challenged these, CHWs were steadfast in their respect of the client's autonomy. These factors are essential to understand how CHWs develop, maintain, and promote positive health outcomes within the moral economy.

The following chapter will shift to explore issues of incorporation experienced by CHWs within the medical and social services workforce. Issues related to the professional incorporation of these workers constructed significant boundaries and barriers for CHWs affecting their ability to perform their duty and ultimately provide caregiving.

NOTES

1. Bourgois 1998, Horton 2015, Nading 2013, Prince 2012.
2. Livingston 2012: 96.
3. Bourgois 1998.
4. Horton 2015.
5. Nading 2013.
6. Lo and Nguyen 2021.
7. Ibid.: 7.
8. Ibid.
9. See, e.g., Marrow 2012, Viladrich 2012.
10. Also known as "white coat hypertension" and refers to patients exhibiting higher than normal blood pressure when visiting a medical professional. However, for the clients of CHWs, this manifested as symptoms of a patient shutting down, feeling condescension from the professional, or without a voice in the appointment.
11. Manson 1988.
12. Blanchard et al. 2007.
13. Ibid.
14. Kumar et al. 2009.
15. Ibid.
16. Traylor et al. 2010.
17. Adams et al. 2015.
18. Schoenthaler et al. 2012.
19. Blanchard et al. 2007.
20. Meghani et al. 2009.
21. See, e.g., Katigbak et al. 2015, Murayama et al. 2017, Wells et al. 2011.
22. Wells et al. 2011.
23. Murayama et al. 2017.
24. Blanchard et al. 2007, Charlot et al. 2015.
25. Sanders et al. 2015.

26. Swartz and Colvin 2015.

27. See, e.g., CHW Central 2017; Closser 2015; U.S. HHS 2007; Maes 2012, 2015a, 2015b, 2016; Maes and Kalofonos 2013; Maes and Shifferaw 2011; Maes et al. 2014; Maes et al. 2015a, 2015b; Ramirez-Valles 1998; Swartz and Colvin 2015.

28. Villa-Torres et al. 2015.

29. Nading 2013.

30. Lo and Nguyen 2021.

Chapter 3

Present Yet Invisible

Issues of Exclusion and Inclusion in the Professional Workforce

"As a doctor . . . I could take out your appendix and it's like 'you're cured!' But when you go home, are you able to get to your next appointment? Get the right foods? Or, what housing do you have to support your needs to keep your health good?" Martha described to me as we discussed the unique roles CHWs fulfill outside of the walls of the clinic. As we continued our conversation, she noted how CHWs can spend significantly more time with clients to ensure health is maintained, a role many medical professionals do not have time for, asserting, "the CHW can get into that [the specific needs of client outside the hospital] because they have the time, whereas the doctor might spend 30, 45 seconds with you and that's pretty much it. They don't know what you need to *maintain* that health." Martha's example highlights just one of the unique roles CHWs can contribute to the established healthcare team (e.g., consisting of medical doctors, nurses, physician associates, social workers, medical assistants). However, until 2017, CHWs in Indiana had never been officially incorporated within the broader, professional workforce despite existing in the state for at least 30 years—emphasizing the present yet invisible nature of this workforce.

Martha expounded on the specific role these workers would play in multi-disciplinary health teams, "That's where I see a great importance for CHWs to be that educator where the doctor or nurse doesn't have time to do that and they're highly paid, they cannot hand hold but the CHW could possibly help that individual and not have them go into relapse." As described throughout the book thus far, the public outreach of these workers fills a gap in care within the United States. Martha noted how these workers help clients and the broader community overcome boundaries and address barriers to care created by lack of access, racism, health inequalities, and other social determinants of health. She further stated, "The CHW could focus on the individual client and help them not go back into the system."

Despite filling many crucial roles, the work of CHWs has gone undervalued and has been largely invisible in Indiana. Moreover, in spite of their significant numbers throughout the state, CHWs remain as largely unknown members of the healthcare workforce with many people in the professional and public realms simply are unaware of what a CHW is and what they do.[1] A variety of factors have instituted boundaries and barriers that hinder the professional integration of these workers including issues related to CHW terminology and a lack of awareness on the part of medical professionals and the general public and a lack of official recognition garnered via certification. While several of the participants were employed within hospitals or clinics, they often went by a different title other than "community health worker." Others found work within the medical field but rather as medical interpreters, and thus were not viewed as a CHW nor could they technically work in such a capacity while on the clock. There is also pushback from accepting them into the healthcare team including from nurses and social workers who are afraid a CHW may replace them. Other times, participants described experiencing condescension from medical professionals when they attended appointments with clients.

Beginning in 2017, steps were being taken by the Community Health Workers' Organization of Indiana (CHWOI), in conjunction with the state government of Indiana, to address these professional issues and fully realize the potential of CHWs. As previously described, the governor of Indiana convened a CHW task force to develop policy, to approve a CHW certification, and to determine a set of CHW-specific, Medicaid reimbursable services. These steps aimed to legitimize these workers in the professional realm and increase their recognition and success. While these official steps are important toward building legitimacy, acceptance, and integration for these workers, they provoke ramifications that must be considered. In this chapter, I explore the various issues that complicate the ability of CHWs to work within the professional realm and assess how professionalization functions as a double-edged sword in increasing their recognition and acceptance.

PROFESSIONAL CITIZENSHIP

As noted in the Introduction, medical citizenship is a theoretical lens defined as "how membership in a state, a society, or even humanity itself is mediated by prevailing regimes of health-related power and knowledge."[2] This framework elucidates whether a population can access health care, health resources, and medical professionals and reveals how individuals and groups do not have equal access to health care and resources.[3] This lens sheds light on a population's belongingness, or citizenship, and thus whether or not this group has a right to health care and is considered morally deserving.[4] The majority of the populations served by CHWs (Black, Asian, Latinx, Indigenous, immigrant, and refugee populations and individuals experiencing homelessness and/or mental and/or substance use disorders) lack medical citizenship due to structural violence, racism, and discrimination. As CHWs typically come from the communities they work within, they too experience the same structural violence and lack of medical citizenship as many of their clients.

As medical citizenship provides a framework for assessing the position of individuals within a society relative to their ability to access care in addition to demonstrating their deservingness of health care, this lens provides insight in revealing how CHWs and their clients were or were not afforded access to care or considered deserving of receiving such resources. Ultimately, this lens highlights how access to care and inclusion (or exclusion) within the healthcare system is operationalized by prevailing regimes of state power.

Additionally, CHWs in Indiana, due to their lack of professional incorporation, experience a kind of workplace structural vulnerability. Participants experienced difficulty in navigating the professional workforce due to lack of recognition, legitimacy, and acceptance that complicated their ability to provide care and procure resources for clients. Much as the state regulates access to care and resources to "deserving" populations and restricting them to those deemed "undeserving," the state, professionals, and employers regulate the ability of CHWs to navigate health and social services and the procurement of resources thereby complicating CHWs' ability to provide care and function to the benefit of their clients and communities.

In this chapter, I utilize the concept of *professional citizenship*, which I define as "the belongingness and legitimacy of a group within the workforce."[5] I draw on this lens in order to elucidate the professional belongingness and acceptance of CHWs within the workforce, including employment within both the medical and social services sectors. This theoretical lens is supported by an additional concept I distinguish as a "legitimizing mechanism," which facilitates professional citizenship. I focus on two primary legitimizing mechanisms: (1) the CHW certification and (2) CHW-specific, Medicaid-reimbursable services. Other legitimizing mechanisms could also include spreading awareness of the CHW model and specialty trainings such as diabetes management, nutrition, doula, midwifery, and other subspecialties.

Certification served as a legitimizing mechanism as it provided a form of "official training" that would allow the CHW to gain a sense of legitimacy when operating in a healthcare environment dominated by advanced degrees, licenses, and registrations (e.g., medical doctor [MD], doctor of osteopathic medicine [DO], physician associate [PA], registered nurse [RN]). Medicaid reimbursement for a set of CHW-specific services also served as a legitimizing mechanism that increased the appeal to hire these workers for employers and potential employers. As reimbursement expands the appeal to hire these workers there is a hope it will result in permanent positions, rather than short-term grant-funded positions, particularly since they provide specific services that are reimbursable via a government agency. Professional citizenship functions as a lens to assess the professional belongingness of CHWs and the legitimizing mechanisms that facilitate their acceptance. In analyzing the specific legitimizing mechanisms, it is possible to identify potential ramifications that may emerge via the process of professionalization, which I detail in the subsequent sections.

The professional citizenship of CHWs is further determined by the ways in which race, gender, and class have been instituted in the professional workforce. The CHW position is an entry-level position in the health care and social services fields and is predominantly made up of women (82% in the United States,[6] an estimated 70% globally,[7] and 80% of participants in this study). Women have also been historically excluded from the professional workforce.[8] Moreover, throughout recent history, women have been largely relegated to auxiliary professions, including dental assistants, nurses, social workers, and midwives, and were further constructed along lines of race, class, and gender.[9] Thus, the lack of professional citizenship experienced by CHWs in Indiana must be understood intersectionally in regards to how factors such as race, class, and gender shape their experience and are (potentially) reproduced through their integration within the workforce.

In the following sections, I detail how CHWs in Indiana encountered variety of obstacles that hindered them from achieving professional citizenship before analyzing how steps were taken to incorporate these workers.

THE TROUBLE WITH TITLES

A major issue that complicated the acceptance and integration for these workers included the extensive titles that fit underneath the "community health worker" umbrella. In my interview with Alisha, we talked at length about the term "community health worker." Alisha described having held many titles but noted that each position was inherently that of a CHW. She told me, "In the past I've been a 'patient navigator,' I've been a 'patient affairs specialist,' I've been a 'community health worker,' I've been a 'family support worker,' I've been a 'health advocate,'" Alisha expounded on the need to have uniformity regarding the title of CHW, asserting "I've been so many things but at the end of the day I get it and we all need to be on one accord about [the term] 'community health worker' because we're here but then you can be a 'health coach' and you don't really know that you really are a community health worker." Alisha stressed the need to create unity with this term to help spread awareness and educate people on what it means to be a community health worker.

The extensive terminology and titles associated with the position served to complicate the public and professional awareness of this position and as a major challenge to the professional citizenship of CHWs. Many participants related to me that the general public seems to have no awareness or clear understanding of what they do. Due to the extensive roles fulfilled by CHWs, which were dependent on the needs of the employer, many of these workers operate under a different title as determined by the employer. Thereby contributing to a lack of awareness of these workers on the part of the public, medical professionals, and potential employers.

At the outset of this research, the Indiana State Department of Health (ISDH) listed 60 terms that fell underneath the umbrella of "community health worker" on their website. I encountered an additional 15 terms during fieldwork and interviews with CHWs. Although these specific titles may come with varying roles and responsibilities, they possess some or all of the characteristics fulfilled by CHWs. The full list of the 75 titles is documented in table 3.1.

Thus, extensive terminology served as a barrier that negatively impacts the professional citizenship of CHWs. It primarily contributes to a lack of awareness regarding what a CHW is and what comprises their responsibilities since the constellation of terms creates confusion and draws attention away from the term "community health worker." In Indiana, as Alisha asserted, the professional workforce and public could become more aware through the use of a singular term.

There are official steps being taken to name brand these various titled positions as "community health worker." Throughout 2017 through 2018, the CHW task force in Indiana—which included Lucía—had drafted a set of certified CHW-specific, Medicaid reimbursable services. The specific language in these billable services includes a provision that they must be performed by a "certified community health worker." As a result, many employers and potential employers will be incentivized to (1) have their employees complete the certification course and (2) change their similarly titled employees to "community health worker" in order to secure reimbursement. Thereby illustrating how certification and Medicaid reimbursable services function as two key legitimizing mechanisms for the professional citizenship of CHWs.

While the institutionalization of the term "community health worker" was seen as necessary (especially due to its usage by the U.S. Bureau of Labor Statistics and mention in the Patient Protection and Affordable Care

Table 3.1 Adapted List of Terms for CHWs from the Indiana State Department of Health

Terms within the CHW Umbrella in Indiana		
Abuse counselor	Family advocate	Medical representative
Access worker	Family education coordinator	Mental health worker
Adult case manager	Family support worker	Natural helper
Assistor	Financial counselor	Navigator
Care coordinator assistant	Health access advocate	Nutrition educator
Care transition coordinator	Health advisor	Outreach advocate
Case coordinator	Health advocate	Outreach case manager
Certified recovery specialist	Health agent	Outreach consultant
Community coordinator	Health assistant	Outreach coordinator
Community counselor	Health broker	Outreach educator
Community health advisor	Healthcare navigator	Outreach worker
Community health coach	Healthcare technician	Parent aide
Community health educator	Health communicator	Parent liaison
Community health representative	Health educator	Patient advocate
Community liaison	Health insurance counselor	Patient navigator
Community organizer	HIV peer advocate	Peer advocate
Community outreach manager	HIV prevention coordinator	Peer leader
Community outreach team force	Home care worker	Peer support coordinator
Community outreach specialist	Home visitor	Peer support specialist
Community outreach worker	Home-based clinician	Promotor/a [de salud]
Community resource liaison	Intake specialist	Roving listener
Community social worker	Interpreter	Rural health access navigator
Discharge planner	Lay health worker	Street outreach worker
Education specialist	Lay health advisor	Youth development specialist
Educator	Maternal and child health case manager	Youth worker

Act [ACA] of 2010), not all of the participants felt this was the best term to capture the services offered by this position. There was division among CHWs about the positive and negative impact in name branding the position as "community health worker." Several participants noted that the legitimacy and name branding as positive benefits related to the CHW position thereby positively contributing to their professional citizenship. Leticia stated, "Especially with the ACA, that first discussion about naming them in the ACA, saying that they could be grant funded. . . . That just gave us the legitimacy. . . . So, we are now at the point where we are right at the opening of the door for health care and community health workers walking through so I'm excited about that." She expanded on how the ACA provides legitimacy as a specific impact of this legislation:

> I think the ACA legitimized [community health workers]. Like I said, it [community health worker position] was before something you named in a grant or whatever, but for some reason when it's a law, when it's something like a federal law especially, it legitimizes the community health worker. And for me it's been a great opportunity for us to say "it's [CHWs] in the ACA, it's a need, we have these health disparities, we have this rising cost of health care, this makes sense." I now have "the word"—as we say in the bible—to preach the word—on community health workers.

Lucía, however, levied a critique of the term "community health worker," explaining, "I don't think it's the best term. Don''t ask me what is the best term [laughter], because it just depends. But I think there is too much health in it . . . and the danger of the term is that it's too medicalized." Lucía recognized that medical issues and access are just part of helping clients and the community achieve well-being. She further explained, "And we know that medical is just a tiny little bit of the person's health. It almost is, 'Well, that's the consequence of everything else that is going on' so we're now calling it the consequence."

Lucía's primary fear is that as the position is legislated and gains Medicaid reimbursement, the foundational aspects of the position such as advocacy and addressing the social determinants of health for clients could be lost in favor of strictly medical-focused activities such as health education, nutrition, and chronic disease management. While these are indeed roles fulfilled by CHWs, Lucía does not want CHWs to lose their ability to advocate and aid clients in the social aspects of health. Other scholars in both public health and anthropology have cautioned how professionalization could provoke fundamental changes to the CHW position including fostering the creation of a CHW hierarchy (enacted through certification, potential for preferential hiring, salary differences based on certification), limiting the scope of abilities of CHWs (i.e., reducing ability to advocate, provide social services), and implementing a credentialing process (i.e., serving as a barrier for entry into the position).[10]

Several participants I spoke with described never having heard of the CHW position prior to attending the certification course. This is reflective of Carla's story described in the previous chapter, in which she had never heard the term before despite working in the same capacity as a CHW. During interviews, I asked participants if they had felt as though they had been doing CHW-like work (prior to knowing the term) and the majority replied that indeed they had been doing this type of work but were unaware there was a term for it. Others had been doing the work of a CHW but had been titled as something else. Similarly, as noted in chapter 2, a few participants felt as though they had been doing this work since childhood either as a volunteer in church activities or in other nongovernmental organizations (NGOs), such as in help-ing immigrant family members navigate bills. Thus, it was possible for par-ticipants to be employed under a different title, though still identifying with the term "community health worker." While terminology presents as a major barrier for the professional citizenship of CHWs, the majority of participants found employment within a variety of settings throughout the state. However, issues persisted in these various areas of employment.

"THE LACK OF KNOWLEDGE": ISSUES FOR CHWS WORKING WITHIN THE BIOMEDICAL REALM

During my time shadowing and interviewing CHWs, many of them spoke to tension they had experienced while either working in or accompanying clients in the biomedical realm. Martha pointed to the fact that the lack of awareness of these workers is at the heart of this tension. She stated, "I would say the lack of knowledge is probably the bigger [issue] and it's not that CHWs are competing with nurses or social workers, in fact they would complement [these workers], but I would say the lack of knowledge is prob-ably the bigger part." As the medical professional was unaware of what a CHW is and why they were present at the appointment, it could result in suspicion, hostility, and condescension aimed at the worker. Relatively, few participants were employed within hospitals and clinics, if they were, they were often employed as a medical interpreter (and rather worked as a CHW clandestinely or after work hours). The primary interactions CHWs had with medical professionals were attending appointments with clients.

Dean explained how declaring "I am a certified community health worker" could result in suspicion and potential condescension. As the medical professional would have no idea who this certified individual is, it would create tension in the medical appointment. During a focus group interview, several CHWs explained they had had to use a different title when advocating for a client in the medical encounter. Brenda, a CHW, explained she has used the term "patient advocate" as a means to try to get doctors to recognize her legitimacy. She explained, "Or even as we call [the patient's medical provider] as their advocate, if you don't have a fancy title they think 'Why should we listen to you?' It can be frustrating when you are talking to the provider and you just need them to open up."

Brenda and Dean's examples highlight how a lack of recognition creates issues in the medical encounter. But a fancy title or lack thereof can lead to suspicion and/or condescension. In either scenario, the lack of recognition of a title and potential for negative interactions underscores the lack of professional citizenship. Moreover, the suspicion on part of the medical professional negatively impacts the potential for a relationship with the CHW. Given that this individual is a nonclinical health worker who interacts with the biomedical environment, other medical professionals may be suspicious of why a CHW should be granted legitimacy within their workplace. Bianca, a Latinx woman and a CHW in her late 20s and employed as a case manager, had worked in both social services organizations and at a volunteer medical clinic. She explained issues she experienced in these environments:

> However, I had both positive and negative interactions with nurses and doctors at our weekend medical clinic. Some were very helpful to me as a community staff member. Another could not believe how little medical knowledge I had, and expected our little, bi-weekly, volunteer-run medical clinic to function very differently. I felt that my studies in a *different* helping profession didn't matter to her, the way she treated me made me feel incompetent.

Bianca's interaction at the volunteer clinic highlights the preconceived notions that medical providers possess about CHWs and what it is exactly they should be doing. Once they had learned of her lack of clinical skills, Bianca's role was devalued by medical professionals. As a result, these professionals delegitimized her place in the medical encounter and further served as a barrier to her professional citizenship.

In October 2017, I spoke with a medical doctor in Indiana who described her work to incorporate CHWs into the broader workforce. Claire explained that she had spent time in an African country collaborating with CHWs to improve health outcomes. Upon returning to Indiana having seen the benefits of CHWs, Claire set out to bring this position to the biomedical realm. She stated, "I was naively surprised initially about some of the pushback [in the U.S.] about having a healthcare provider who didn't have a certification and a preexisting stamp of approval." Claire elaborated that she did not encounter this resistance during her work abroad due to the overwhelming need for health workers in general.

Although participants explained how a lack of awareness and/or condescension has served as a barrier that highlights their lack of professional citizenship, they expounded that medical professionals typically responded well to the work of CHWs once they had learned more about their roles.

Rosa, a Latinx woman, CHW, and doula with over 20 years of experience, explained that at first, doctors were skeptical of her role but later came to appreciate her skills. Rosa also spent time locating and providing peer-reviewed studies regarding doulas and their efficacy in order to provide medical professionals with further reasons to justify her professional citizenship. Andrés had similar experiences in his work with medical professionals. He typically spends half his day as a medical interpreter and the other half conducting community outreach. Andrés explained how doctors and other medical professionals were very receptive to him in both of these roles:

> In fact, they are very grateful to have somebody and not just because of the interpreter, [to address] the language barrier, but the way that they communicate effectively with the patient and also, even as a community health worker, they know that we are a very good resource because sometimes they have to see a patient that needs to see a specialist. For example, an oncologist, and in the right moment they [the doctors] know of several oncologists *pero* [but] they know they are very expensive and sometimes they ask me "do you know any kind of resources like that?" I'll go "yeah, I know somebody, a doctor that they can offer even some way for them to pay their bill even in installment or maybe they have financial assistance and I even have those forms already." And they just kind of say "Oh really?! That's great, can you help them with that?" And I say "Sure, I can help them with that." So yes, the physicians they feel really comfortable and I know they are grateful and also, we are thankful for their services that they can count on the community health worker to even facilitate their job with this community.

As Andrés and Rosa's examples demonstrate, once doctors learned more about their roles and services they provide, the more willing they seemed to have CHWs as part of the healthcare team, thereby removing this professional barrier that impeded these workers from being part of the team. I should, however, note that Andrés dualistic role of a medical interpreter *and* CHW was the exception rather than the norm in the case of Indiana. The majority of CHWs employed within the biomedical realm worked solely as medical interpreters and were, technically, unable to perform any roles as a CHW. While these individuals were still personally considered themselves as a CHW, they were unable to use this title in their employment. As a result, this contributed to the overarching problem regarding lack of recognition and awareness of the CHW title. This lack of recognition within the professional medical workforce was understood by participants as a major problem hindering their ability to attain professional citizenship.

PROFESSIONAL CITIZENSHIP AS A MEDICAL
INTERPRETER BUT NOT AS A CHW

The majority of participants who had employment in a medical environment worked as medical interpreters officially, rather than a CHW. As noted earlier, however, as medical interpreters, participants encountered a barrier that restricted the services they could provide. Their sole responsibility was to interpret, word-for-word, between doctor and patient. Thus, all roles as a CHW had to be set aside until they were off the clock. I detail in the following chapter the struggles these participants faced that, at times, forced them to go outside of their scope of care as interpreters. This demarcation between these two positions served to the detriment of participants, with many lamenting that this left their full potential as CHWs unrealized.

One participant explained, as I shadowed her at a volunteer clinic that, in her medical interpreting job, she is only allowed to translate and was required to leave the room if the doctor left the room. Carmen, as noted earlier was a *promotora* by title, explained how she advocates for the patient regardless of her role to strictly translate as a medical interpreter. As previously noted, Carmen was unique among CHWs in that she had a PhD and had previously worked as a scientist. She pondered how a "real" *promotora* would handle interactions with medical professionals given that this individual would not have the training and perhaps lack the confidence that comes with a PhD. Additionally, complications arose in this situation since the job position "*promotora*/CHW" is not well-recognized nor understood at her hospital. And, despite her title and advocacy work, she is not viewed as a *promotora* but rather as a medical interpreter since medical professionals interact with her mostly in this role.

Additional boundaries and barriers emerged regarding the professional citizenship of CHWs when they served in the capacity of an interpreter due to medical professionals and hospital staff viewing them solely as interpreters and not as CHWs. While these "interpreter-CHWs" described experiencing a positive relationship with the medical provider, the majority of whom were happy to have them there to translate, this was the only legitimacy they could claim—as medical interpreters, *not* as CHWs. As noted earlier, medical professionals were sometimes suspicious or condescending toward CHWs who accompanied clients to appointments and spoke up on their behalf rather than just interpreting. This caused CHWs to use a different term to justify speaking up for the patient during the interaction and justify their inclusion. Since some participants stated that the term "community health worker" either did not "make sense" to medical professionals (due to lack of recognition of this title) or it could be understood as "threatening." Thus, professional citizenship was attained while serving as an interpreter but was lost if serving in the role of a CHW.

Ultimately, reconciling these two job categories could address some issues in terms of professional citizenship. While an interpreter might be a CHW, it does not mean they have the same training. The role of the interpreter could be expanded to allow those who are also trained as CHWs to help patients address the social determinants of health and ensure their needs are met outside of the doctor's appointment. As will be discussed further in the following chapter, interpreter-CHWs, such as Carmen, would speak up for clients during interpreting but also provide clients with her contact information clandestinely in order to extend additional services as a CHW.

CHALLENGES IN SOCIAL SERVICE AND
COMMUNITY-BASED ORGANIZATIONS

Many participants, and CHWs in general, work in social service agencies or community-based organizations. While these CHWs still accompanied clients to medical appointments or worked as interpreters, they were not employed by a clinic or hospital. CHWs employed in these organizations still encountered boundaries related to their professional citizenship, not from their employer but rather during encounters with medical professionals. Many of the participants employed in these organizations were termed as something else, typically a title that fit the needs of the organization. Other issues they encountered included challenges such as tenuous funding for their position, which was often secured through short-term grants that lasted only one to several years, barring the employing organization receiving additional funding. This tenuous funding was a key concern related to the sustainability of such a position.

Participants also encountered similar issues with terminology and job as their counterparts in the biomedical realm. CHWs working in social services organizations were typically titled differently than "community health worker," which served as a barrier in their interaction with other professionals (see table 3.1). Participants that worked in social service agencies or community-based organizations explained that they also would use the term "patient advocate" in an attempt to gain some legitimacy in their encounters with medical professionals and other organizations. While some professionals seemed to understand and be receptive to this term, it limited the broader awareness of the term "community health worker." Lucía, a CHW and had recently trained as a chaplain, explained,

I deal a lot with patients in the hospital and palliative care . . . most of my personal connection with them [medical professionals] is coming in [the hospital] and they don't understand when I tell them I'm their [the patient's] "community health worker," they understand when I tell them I'm their "patient advocate." And when I tell them I'm a patient advocate, everything changes. They really share information with the patient there, they are more willing to explain in more detail their procedures or their care plan, but I'm usually dealing with the physicians when they come in and they talk to our patients . . .but yeah, it's "patient advocate" is what I have to throw out there or "chaplain" and then they open up. But if I say "CHW" they just say ". . . Ok."

Lucía's example again emphasizes the problems related to terminology related to the CHW title and how it is not well-understood or even accepted within this environment. She was only granted information regarding her client when the medical professional in the encounter understands her role as a "patient advocate" or "chaplain," despite the former essentially being another term for community health worker. Thus, in spite of official designations of the title "community health worker" in the U.S. Bureau of Labor Statistics and in the ACA, there is still little recognition and reticence toward accepting the position as a part of the healthcare team thereby impeding the professional citizenship of these workers.

CHWS AS VOLUNTEERS

Only five of the participants functioned in the role of a CHW solely as a volunteer. Although it was common among the sample for CHWs to work as a volunteer while off the clock, several participants had specific reasons for performing this work on a volunteer basis. One participant, Ximena, who several months before our interview had completed the certification course, wanted to be employed as a CHW but was unable to find paid work in this position. As a result, she found employment within the insurance industry. Ximena told me that although she is not employed as a CHW, she draws on her training when helping clients in her job and also participates when she is able to in community events as a volunteer CHW. The lack of CHW positions thus forces some to work in this capacity solely in their free time.

Other participants served as volunteers because they were integrating their work as a CHW within their daily work life. Alejandra had previously completed an internship with the Mexican consulate in Indianapolis but had since become a stay-at-home mom. However, she is an active volunteer within the Latinx community in Indianapolis, serving community members by connecting them to resources, as a health educator, and in various other community issues. Valentina, an owner of a childcare business and CHW, told me that she integrates her training as a CHW within her business. She connects the parents of the children in her daycare with resources and other health services as needed. Magdalena, a middle-aged Latinx woman and an ESL teaching assistant who had also completed the CHW training, volunteers with an immigrant advocacy center in Indianapolis and helps to connect clients with any services they need.

While employed full-time in various other professions, these participants served as volunteer CHWs in and outside of their employment. Although providing services as a volunteer CHW fills important gaps in care to clients and the community, it also demonstrates how the position is not viewed as a legitimate job due to the lack of employers hiring CHWs (in addition to the tenuous, short-term-funded positions described in the previous section). However, there are steps being taken to increase the number of employers hiring CHWs and to improve their professional citizenship and inclusion in the workforce.

BUILDING PROFESSIONAL CITIZENSHIP

A variety of pieces must come together in order for CHWs to be incorporated successfully as a member of the professional workforce. Steps taken by policy-makers include policy development (including approving the CHW certification and CHW-specific Medicaid reimbursement) to demonstrate official, state government acceptance of this position. The certification provides reassurance to the professional community of a foundational level training and a "new" title of "certified community health worker" (CCHW, thereby also providing a set of letters to follow a name, much as doctors and nurses have MD and RN, respectively). Scholars have asserted that CHW certification could provide job security, increase recognition, and standardize the workforce.[11] Medicaid reimbursement provides an economic justification for hiring CHWs, due to their ability to be reimbursed for CHW-specific services. While Indiana has taken steps in both developing policy for Medicaid reimbursement and state-supported certification, the effects of these steps on the professional citizenship of the CHW workforce in Indiana remains to be seen.

Aside from the professional citizenship needed by CHWs within the workforce, their communities must also be connected to and considered deserving of care. Many participants and CHWs overall come from marginalized populations. As CHWs, they face a need for double legitimacy since the majority also share the structural vulnerability of their clients. Steps at the policy level should be taken to provide medical citizenship to their communities—and as an additional means to address health disparities and social determinants of health. These topics were echoed during the photovoice project. Gabriela, a

CHW who comes from and works within the Latinx immigrant community, lamented that she has had to overcome a challenge in that not everyone is included in the American Dream. She took the following photograph and captioned it, "Overcoming the idea that the Land of Opportunity is for everyone" (see figure 3.1).

She expounded on the caption and photograph, specifically describing the challenges faced by her community and immigrants that made her reassess her understanding of the supposed values and symbolism of the United States. Gabriela stated, "I mean there's that belief when they [immigrants] first arrive that this is the land of opportunity and they're going to help me and then you realize 'well, you're not documented so we can't really help you.'" She continued, "And when you have kids or people that are adults that are suicidal, while you can take them in for an assessment anywhere [and] do the assessment, but then there's no treatment because they don't qualify. To me . . . it's hard to overcome that idea."

The surfeit of resources available in Indiana added to her, and other photovoice participants', dejected feelings of disillusionment regarding the United States. These feelings, coupled with the wealth of the United States, made it hard for her to accept that an individual could be evaluated for a mental health

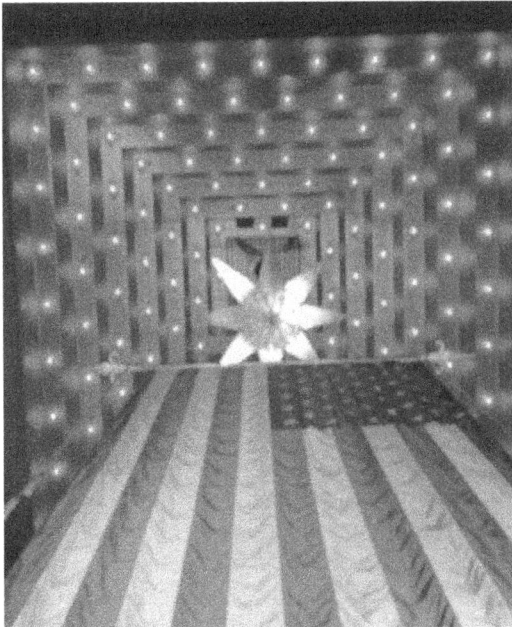

Figure 3.1   "Overcoming the idea that the Land of Opportunity is for everyone."
Source: Photo by Gabriela (Pseudonym).

disorder and still be denied treatment due to their immigration or financial status despite the resource being available. Her example highlights the shared structural vulnerability of the CHW and their clients. Although Gabriela is in a better position financially and health-wise, she is unable to help her clients fully access certain resources depending on their legal and financial status. Thus, wider systemic changes must occur to ensure the medical citizenship of these populations and address issues of inclusion for CHWs within the workforce.

OPENING THE DOOR: CERTIFICATION AS A MEANS TO PROVIDE LEGITIMACY AND INCLUSION

I first learned of the state-supported CHW certification during my pilot research in 2016. The certification was developed in partnership with a nonprofit health organization headquartered in the Midwest in addition to heavy involvement with CHWOI. Among the supporters of the development of this certification included the ISDH. At the beginning of data collection in June 2017, CHWOI had received a substantial grant to train 100 CHWs and help them find employment as CCHWs. The certification would serve as a legitimizing mechanism to help these workers attain professional citizenship. Certification also serves as a means to increase job security, recognition, and standardization of the CHW workforce.[12]

The lack of certification served as a predominant barrier for these workers from locating employment and acceptance within the workforce. Potential employers, especially in the medical workforce, have been hesitant to employ an individual without some type of "formal" training. While CHWs are certainly educated in health and social issues, with many taking workshops or specialty trainings, these had not been sufficient to find gainful or at least stable employment. Moreover, many CHWs, in terms of education, may not have more than a high school degree, further hampering their ability to gain employment. This certification would address these issues and serve as a type of degree to provide legitimacy for these workers.

While various training and certification courses exist for CHWs throughout the United States, in Indiana the certification provides these workers with a new title, "certified community health worker" (CCHW), and was established to provide new avenues into the professional workforce. Importantly, this certification also serves as the direct connection for receiving Medicaid reimbursement. Employees would need to complete the certification and earn the CCHW title to qualify for reimbursement thereby reinforcing the certification's status as a primary legitimizing mechanism.

Many participants described the positive impacts that certification produced. Victoria, a CHW of five months' experience, stated that with the certification she felt more qualified to do the work, boosted her self-confidence, and made her motivated to keep up with the qualifications of being a CHW. Clark, a White man in his 40s and CHW with four years of experience, explained to me that he felt it provided more "credence" to medical providers to partner with CHWs. Leticia explained how the certification provides legitimacy for CHWs within the workforce, stating,

The certification of the community health worker brings . . . legitimacy and I know that sometimes they're opening doors for our residents and community that normally they cannot open for themselves. I'll let you know right now that if the community health worker calls, they are more likely to get through than if some resident calls in and says "I want to talk to the doctor or I want to talk to the nurse." "This is so-and-so from [an employing organization], I am a community health worker . . . " it opens the door. It opens the door for an appointment, it opens the door for if there is an emergency, it opens the door. So, having the certification in the title I think it is going to open doors and help the community. It's somebody legitimate from the *community* and it's not somebody from the healthcare system . . . they [CHWs] are very strong leaders . . . and they are leaders not just as a community health worker, they are leaders in various areas like in immigration, they are leaders in the lead crisis,[13] so having community health workers embedded or being part of all of the settings of what is going on in the community is a great opportunity.

Carmen also echoed these sentiments in gaining additional legitimacy as a result of the certification as well as getting her employers to expand her role as a medical interpreter to be inclusive of her skills as a CHW. Carmen spoke fondly of the certification course, the skills she learned, and how the certification itself has provided her with another tool to sell the benefits of being a CHW. She stated,

What this training helped me so much with . . . [is being able to] sell this idea of being a CHW, say to a hospital board. And it [the certification] really does help when you have to deal with some of these doctors. I get them when I come in and I'm just somebody that speaks Spanish. Every now and then they [medical professionals] try to blind somebody with science and I lay some back on 'em and it's like "Oh boy . . ." All of a sudden they cool their jets and start speaking plain English, so I can speak plain Spanish so the patient understands. Now with the CHW training I can say "Would you like me to see if this person gets on Medicaid" or whatever, and it's like "You can do that?" and I say, "I can find it out." That's some of the things I feel like I can take it another step. And now I think most of them listen to me, it's a huge respect level back from the medical professionals who consider us just again somebody's grandma or kid that's in there speaking Spanish [and] that helps tremendously.

In spite of the legitimacy that certification affords there is the chance for ramifications, which may exclude some from becoming CHWs. The grant received by CHWOI provided tuition-waivers for 100 CHWs but now that the grant has ended, the cost may be insurmountable for some. Especially as many CHWs come from underserved and impoverished communities, they may be unable to take time off work (the certification is a 70-hour training) and/or afford to pay the cost of the class ($1,500). To address these issues, the course has been offered in alternate schedules (e.g., staggered over a month), with financial support via scholarships and employer-paid tuition, and implementing a grandfathering process for CHWs with extensive experience.[14] However, the cost and time needed to complete the course may remain as a barrier for some.

Other participants were ambivalent about the actual impact the certification had on their work as a CHW. Participants who had extensive experience as a CHW felt particularly undecided about the impact of certification. While many felt it had enhanced and reinforced their skillset, the training did little to teach them something new. Amanda stated, "Honestly, I don't think that it's even impacted me that much. But it's nice having more of a label and a training behind it. But I don't think that it made any of my qualities stronger or more recognizable." I then asked if she felt if the training instead just reinforced her existing skills and knowledge. She responded, "Yeah. I think just being able to tell people I'm a 'certified community health worker' makes them feel a little bit better about who they are interacting with." Thus, regardless of specific technical insights, the certification still made participants feel as those they might secure professional citizenship as a "certified" community health worker.

Aside from CHWs, other stakeholders described the benefits of certification but also cautioned that it can be a double-edged sword. In my conversations with Claire, she argued that "certification is . . . a double-edged sword. . . . Certifying implies something else . . . if it's in health care you have to certify because everybody in health care has to be certified one way or another." Claire also expounded on the legitimacy it can afford, "So that [certification] legitimizes that [CHWs] within the context of the healthcare system. But what does that mean to a social service agency and what does that mean to the community itself? So I don't see it as one level, I think there's going to be certification that's going to be needed and required from the healthcare setting."

These examples demonstrate how the certification provides legitimacy but can also result in ramifications. For CHWs who are undocumented, they may be unable to pay for the training or may encounter a language barrier as the course is currently only offered in English (although the grant provided a free ESL course for those needing additional help with their English language ability). Even if they are able to attain the certification, they will be unable to be hired in the majority of cases due to their legal status. The certification course may also exclude those who do not perform well in a classroom environment. Furthermore, depending on how the CHW model is professionalized, there is the chance that the foundation of the position may be changed in order to appease employers and/or medical professionals. Examples of this include reducing the ability of CHWs to advocate, preventing CHWs from spending time helping clients to overcome social determinants of health, and/or overmedicalizing their responsibilities—especially in terms of what services are dictated to be reimbursable via Medicaid.

I spoke extensively with Martha about the potential ramifications that could be invoked. Martha told me, "I think eventually, in reality, that the certification will take precedence, not that the ones without cannot get a job, but I feel that at some point the certification, like a degree, at some point it's going to take precedence over an employer saying 'Ok, because this means that this person has been formally trained and passed some kind of an exam.'" However, she was quick to point out that this certification should not (and, ideally, will not) preclude noncertified CHWs from still having a role to fill in other organizations. Martha elaborated, "Not that, there will still be places in the community, the churches, and so forth for those that may not hold it [the certification] but I would say for many of the upper level or higher positions in organizations and companies, I feel personally that the certification is going to move up."

While the benefits and complications of certification are still being negotiated in Indiana, there is a general consensus, especially, among those involved in the professionalization of the CHW position that the benefits outweigh potential complications. CHWs have been largely stuck in limbo and have faced a variety of barriers such as invisible to general public, potential employers, and medical professionals despite being present in the state for decades and in urban and rural communities in Indiana. Certification, at the moment, is viewed as a necessary legitimizing mechanism despite its inherent status as a double-edged sword. This legitimizing mechanism can produce increased awareness and acceptance, thereby leading to professional citizenship for CHWs. However, it will be vital that CHWs are included in conversations about the professional development of their position and granted control over its direction.

MEDICAID REIMBURSEMENT
AS A LEGITIMIZING MECHANISM

Directly connected to certification and as an equally important legitimizing mechanism is Medicaid reimbursement for a set of CHW-specific services. Ideally, this will increase the appeal of hiring CHWs throughout the state. Throughout 2017 and 2018, along with the development of the CHW position, officials from the Office of Medicaid Policy and Planning worked to draft a set of billable services. These services included CHW instruction of self-management training and health education. While these are important roles fulfilled by CHWs, the billable services were written to exclude reimbursement for enrollment assistance, case management, or advocacy.

With the advent of the ACA, scholars have noted how Medicaid reimbursement for CHW services has expanded potential.[15] Among some of the provisions in the ACA for CHWs includes states being given the authority to designate non-licensed providers that can give preventative services.[16] Other states have already provided Medicaid reimbursement for CHW services including Arizona, Minnesota, and Oregon.[17] Minnesota, in particular, is a case in which there is an established funding stream for these workers and a wide range of CHW-specific reimbursable services have helped realize a broader potential for these workers.[18]

However, Lucía was critical of the finalized set of reimbursable services, primarily because they were strictly medically focused and did not provide reimbursement for time spent addressing social determinants of health. Thus, activities that address the environmentally determined aspects of health, such as helping clients overcome social determinants of health, could be diminished or lost entirely in favor of services that are reimbursable. While Lucía continues to advocate during policy development for the adoption of a broader set of reimbursable services, as of 2021, they remain the same.

While the finalized set of reimbursable services left much to be desired, it remains as a legitimizing mechanism for the professional citizenship of CHWs. However, as the noted services are strictly health-focused, this may shift the roles and responsibilities of these workers. Undoubtedly, current and potential employers will prioritize their CHWs to perform tasks that are reimbursable thereby diminishing their ability to perform activities such as advocacy.[19] This would likely shift the foundation of the CHW model in Indiana—many participants described how advocacy and helping clients address that the social determinants of health was the cornerstone of their caregiving.

Additionally, as Medicaid reimbursement provides an additional incentive to hire CHWs, it is possible they will need to produce positive outcomes for the bottom line of the budget for their employing organization. Participants noted that despite being able to provide reimbursable services, they will likely not see their pay increase. Carmen explained that she will likely still be underpaid even if her employer is able to save money as a result of reimbursement, highlighting structural racism and the gender pay gap in addition to how the neoliberal economic model is integrated into the ramifications of introducing CHWs into the workforce.[20] Thus, Medicaid reimbursement serves as a legitimizing mechanism but provokes potential ramifications—increased inclusion and professional citizenship in exchange for a diminished ability to participate in crucial roles fulfilled by the CHW model.

MOVING FORWARD: CHWS AS MEMBERS OF THE MULTIDISCIPLINARY HEALTHCARE TEAM

Ideally, the aforementioned legitimizing mechanisms, including certification and Medicaid reimbursement, will integrate CHWs as an official member of the healthcare team. Participants were also keenly aware of some of the gaps CHWs could fulfill if better incorporated within the workforce. Other participants, especially those who are managing other CHWs or who have worked with developing the CHW certification, asserted that CHWs are in a similar position to the one nurse practitioners and physician associates were before they became accepted members of the healthcare team. Marcia, a CHW and a director of a health outreach program, explained,

> But we do probably see it [pushback from medical professionals regarding CHWs] coming, especially when you start placing [the CHWs in jobs]. It probably is very similar to when nurse practitioners came on board and when physician assistants came on board and how the doctors challenged those. And then they saw, "Oh, these are valuable people, you know, there are some things they can do that I don't have to do that anymore." And then you find out that a lot of people that used to go to their doctor say, "Oh, I'd rather talk to the nurse practitioner." So, I'm sure that as time progresses, we will see that. We are hoping it will be a team effort so it won't be just "you don't value me as a community health worker." So, we are looking at a team approach.

In spite of evidence found in the academic literature regarding the real (and potential) successes CHWs may have if inducted into the healthcare team, Lucía still saw this as coalescing further into the future rather than sooner. She explained to me that she still thinks Indiana is four to five years away from a strong CHW presence in the workforce, stating, "It almost feels very territorial that the medical community does not want to add a new member to the team and very shortsighted. I think those two things really get in the way of the movement and I see that when those things go away in other states that there's an openness to CHWs on the team."

Until this openness is fostered by the broader professional community and potential employers, CHWs in Indiana will lack professional citizenship and, thereby, face perpetual boundaries. This acceptance can be garnered as several participants described working in partnerships with nurses or on small, informal teams with medical doctors at free clinics. These participants described positive experiences working in this capacity as a team. Previous research has also demonstrated positive outcomes with CHWs in collaborative teams.[21] Wider acceptance of CHWs as a new member of the healthcare team could strengthen the broader healthcare workforce and bring about positive health impacts for the whole of the state—and build the professional citizenship of CHWs.

UNCLOAKING THE ROLE OF
CHWS IN THE WORKFORCE

There is a variety of moving pieces to consider when assessing how CHWs are excluded and how steps toward inclusion of the CHW model within the professional workforce in Indiana will affect the profession. These workers have been without professional citizenship and also share structural vulnerability along with their clients and communities. Participants described similar professional challenges despite being employed in different settings. Extensive terminology and the lack of recognition on part of the public and professionals in conjunction with suspicion and condescension for their presence in the medical encounter spurned the ability of CHWs to gain acceptance in the workforce. However, the state government and CHWOI have worked toward professionalizing CHWs to enhance their legitimacy and acceptance in the professional workforce.

Several steps are and can be taken in order to foster greater professional citizenship for CHWs in Indiana and provide them with bridges across these boundaries. These include certification, Medicaid reimbursement, and acceptance by professionals in the workforce. Moreover, via certification and reimbursement, the myriad of titles will be replaced with "community health worker" as the official title thereby addressing the issue of extensive terminology. While each of these can be a double-edged sword, they are noted by many participants as necessary steps toward official incorporation into the workforce and, ideally, secure professional citizenship.

Furthermore, understanding the intersectional impacts of race, gender, ethnicity, and class regarding their institutionalization within the professional workforce is crucial as CHWs undergo professionalization.[22] These sociodemographic factors have placed women and, particularly, women of color at a disadvantage complicated their acceptance into the workforce and resulted in pay disparities in the professional realm. Understanding how these structural forces are operationalized and reproduced at the professional level is pivotal to ensure equitable acceptance of these workers going forward.

CHWs must maintain ownership of the direction of their profession as steps are taken regarding its professionalization and be included in any discussion of their incorporation, including how it will affect their roles, responsibilities, and future direction of their profession.[23] The American Public Health Association's Community Health Worker Section[24] and Sabo et al.[25] assert that CHWs must make up at least 50 percent of the representation of legislation developed regarding their position. Specifically, the APHA and Sabo et al. argue that this will provide CHWs with the much-needed control over the direction of their job. Alisha summed up this issue in Indiana during our interview, stating,

> I don't think that upper people need to be creating this [policy development regarding the CHW model]. We need to have community health workers right at the table. You . . . need more than one [CHW on the task force]. It should be structured half and half, or a third. You have some [policy makers], you have some medical management people, you have some social work people, you have a couple CHWs that are doing different things. Mix it up.

While steps are being taken to professionalize and provide professional citizenship for these workers, CHWs are faced with challenging situations that enact boundaries and barriers—situations in which they must decide to remain within their scope of care or step outside it. Chapter 4 takes a deeper look at several boundaries encountered by CHWs and how their roles and responsibilities are situated in a gray area in terms of caregiving. Although steps at greater incorporation of these workers may address some of these issues, it may be that this scope of care that exists in a gray area yields positive health outcomes for the clients of CHWs.

NOTES

1. Sherwen et al. 2007.
2. Good et al. 2010: 177.
3. Goldade 2009, Good et al. 2010, Nichter 2008, Wailoo et al. 2006.
4. Goldade 2009.
5. Logan 2021, 194.
6. U.S. HHS 2007.

7. CHW Central 2017.

8. Witz 1992.

9. Adams 1998; Butler, Chillas, and Muhr 2012; Dahle 2012; Witz 1992.

10. Arvey and Fernandez 2012, Bovbjerg et al. 2013, Catalani et al. 2009, Maupin 2011, Nading 2013.

11. Ingram et al. 2020.

12. Ibid.

13. This region of Indiana continues to experience issues with lead in the drinking water, see https://www.chicagotribune.com/suburbs/post-tribune/ct-ptb-east-chicago -one-year-later-st-0723-20170721-story.html.

14. In August 2020, CHWOI began grandfathering CHWs as certified community health workers. Several requirements were developed to be eligible, including: being 18 years or older; have a high school diploma/GED equivalent or higher degree; must be a U.S. citizen or permanent resident of Indiana (or a bordering state); worked or volunteer 4,000 hours providing CHW services within the past five years; and provide three letters of recommendation.

15. George et al. 2020, Katzen and Morgan 2014, Rosenthal et al. 2010, Schmit et al. 2021.

16. Katzen and Morgan 2014.

17. George et al. 2020, Ingram et al. 2020, Rosenthal et al. 2010.

18. Rosenthal et al. 2010.

19. Nading 2013, Pérez and Martinez 2008.

20. Logan 2021.

21. See, e.g., Allen et al. 2014, Deitrick et al. 2010, Enard and Ganelin 2013, Findley et al. 2014, Walton et al. 2012.

22. Butler, Chillas, and Muhr 2012; Dahle 2012; Witz 1992.

23. APHA 2014, Catalani et al. 2009, Closser et al. 2019, C3 2018, Ingram et al. 2020, Pérez and Martinez 2008, Rosenthal et al. 2011, Sabo et al. 2013.

24. APHA 2014.

25. Sabo et al. 2015.

Chapter 4

Boundaries of Care

How Caregiving Is Shaped in Community Health Work

"As we are waiting in the appointment, I'm asking her other things, 'Do you have enough food? Because I'm a volunteer at a local food bank. And I'm sitting there like, 'Well, I could take you over there later,'" Carmen recounted her conversation with a client while waiting for the doctor to enter the room. As previously discussed, Carmen is a medical interpreter but also trained as a CHW. However, officially, in this appointment, she was serving as a medical interpreter and not in her role as a *promotora*. Carmen continued, "So, as an interpreter I'm violating all kinds of things, advocacy and chatting about everything outside [of the appointment]. But I do wear many hats." For Carmen, this violation of working in the capacity as a CHW while interpreting was morally justified to ensure the patient would be fully cared for. Technically, in her role as an interpreter she is to remain solely as a mouthpiece—translating, word-for-word, between the medical professional and the patient. However, this was extremely frustrating to Carmen who argued there is much more she can offer to ensure that the patient receives the needed care, resources, and services.

Healthcare professionals follow a scope of care (also known as "scope of practice"), which outlines their professional responsibilities, capacities, and other factors that dictate their ability to provide care. This scope of care establishes boundaries for the CHW to adhere to when providing care and engaging with clients. The Community Health Workers' Organization of Indiana (CHWOI) outlines their scope of care as the roles and core competencies in the certification course (see table 0.1 in the Introduction). For CHWs in Indiana, their scope of care broadly includes maintaining a professional relationship with clients and adhering to the CHW core responsibilities and tenets. There are also scopes of care defined at the national level, within the state, outlined in the certification course, and possible additional scopes of care mandated by employer expectations and/or based on specialty trainings (e.g., doula, midwifery, chronic disease management, etc.) that the CHW may have completed. However, many participants, at particular times, went outside of their scope of care in order to provide a necessary service for their client—driven by their moral obligation to provide the best possible care and resources—thereby justifying crossing the boundaries established by the scope of care.

Carmen continued, "To me, in the ideal *promotora* program, I would have to address that [the other needs of the client] because if she is not eating the right food as a diabetic that's why the wound is not healing, that's why the kidneys are failing, I get it . . . and I've gone through all these steps. I've since had to take her to the kidney people." In her example, Carmen makes the conscious decision to cross boundaries of care that are defined by the scope of care of medical interpretation to provide the services of a CHW. Carmen is fortunate in that she works part-time and has retired following a long career as a scientist and can thus take risks in crossing these boundaries. Nonetheless, it is a choice that many participants had to make and justify either remaining within designated guidelines or crossing them in pursuit of the best care possible for their clients.

This was especially true when it came to advocating for the needs of the patient. Carmen stated, "I'm not supposed to do that [advocate] as an interpreter, that's one of my faults [laughter]. I advocate for my doctor [who] prescribed something and I bring up, 'Is this going to be costly?' Because this patient is a total charity care thing." However, in stepping outside of the scope of care for medical interpreters, Carmen enhanced the collaboration between the medical professional and patient in ensuring that the medication was affordable and social determinants of health that could impede adherence to the treatment plan are understood and addressed. Regardless of the potential ethical (and legal) dilemmas that could be encountered as a result of going outside of the designated scope of care, Carmen morally justified crossing this boundary in order to provide adequate care for her client.

In exploring how CHWs approach their caregiving, it is vital to assess how legislators and other stakeholders shape, define, and enact barriers and boundaries related to how these workers provide care. These boundaries take the form of laws, policies, regulations, scope of care, and funding that impact the ability of CHWs to provide care and operate effectively in their role. While essentially all of these laws, policies, and regulations are developed without the input of CHWs, they have massive impacts on the environment in which CHWs operate and navigate the moral economy of care. Moreover, as chapter 3 established, CHWs lack professional citizenship which further complicates their ability to operate within the biomedical and public arenas. While more recent steps are being taken, which include some input from CHWs in terms of the professionalization of their position, CHWs are still faced with a variety of boundaries and barriers as they provide care.

Policies, laws, regulations, and the certification process also affect the ability of CHWs to provide care and specifically challenge these workers to remain within their established scope of care. Participants described being faced staying within or going outside these scopes of care depending on the needs of the client. Assessing how these laws, policies, and practices—especially for medical paraprofessionals such as CHWs—is essential to understand how they shape care and the relationship between these workers and clients.[1] Aside from the imperative to enact laws on the part of legislators, CHWs—as noted in chapters 1 and 2—are motivated by their own morality, which, in turn, strongly impacts the provision of their caregiving and intimately shapes their relationships and obligations in the moral economy of care. In this chapter, I explore how CHWs encountered barriers and boundaries in caregiving and the decisions they made to cross or stay within these guidelines.

CONSTRUCTING BOUNDARIES OF CAREGIVING AND ENACTING CHALLENGES VIA POLICY

In order to set the stage for how the caregiving of CHWs was shaped, I detail several federal and state laws, policies, and programs that impacted the care and established specific boundaries and barriers. CHWs encountered these as they provided care and at times were boundaries to be crossed while at other times were barriers that prevented the procurement of resources or further caregiving.

The Patient Protection and Affordable Care Act of 2010 (ACA)

The ACA was a landmark law passed in 2010 that has had substantial impact in providing insurance to Americans, especially among people of color.[2] Aside from significantly reducing rates of uninsured, parts of the law recognized CHWs by name and outlined several opportunities for these workers—including potential funding streams.[3] The ACA and its impacts on subsequent laws and programs passed at the state level created significant impacts for CHWs and their clients. When I asked participants what the impact of the ACA has been, many responded that it has produced positive outcomes for their clients. Some CHWs trained as ACA navigators to help clients sign up for health insurance and as an additional means of employment. Other participants noted that many of their clients attained health insurance through the Medicaid expansion as part of the ACA.[4] Thus, for many of the clients of CHWs, the ACA removed barriers that prevented access to care for many of their clients and, thereby, reshaped the healthcare landscape that CHWs operate within.

However, when I asked if the ACA has had any impacts on the CHW position itself, the majority of the participants responded that it has made no difference at all. This was unsurprising given that the CHW funding streams initially set up in the ACA never materialized. Leticia argued that the ACA codified CHWs in providing name branding and legitimacy noted in chapter 3, other participants were not so sure. Lucía offered a more nuanced take on the specific impacts that the ACA had on both CHWs and their clients. Although she recognized the importance of mentioning these workers by title in the legislation, she also noted that the law has had negative impacts on some populations:

> It [the ACA] has also been negative in that it's caused some health care to go away for some of our populations. People become more aware—well, health care being available for individuals who are undocumented. Now that there's a way for hospital and clinics for measuring their effectiveness and so what that's done is almost like the collateral damage is because these individuals are "high-risk" or "noncompensative"—there's no way to get compensation by treating them—then we won't treat them. So that's been a common thing to happen with a lot of healthcare systems . . . they become collateral damage, so that would be the one thing that is negative. But creating awareness for the profession has been good so it's kind of been both [positive and negative].

While she felt overall that the name branding within the ACA contributed to the recognition of CHWs—and thereby their professional citizenship—she also described the boundaries placed by the official recognition of the title itself. She asserted, "The problem with name branding something like that [CHW] is that if it doesn't fit, people just can't figure out how to [use it]—it's too rigid. It would have been better to mention it [CHW position] by function, 'the functions provided by these individuals, otherwise known as CHWs . . .' that would have been much better." Thus, Lucía argued that the ACA could have left more flexibility related to the wording in the law when it came to utilizing and implementing the CHW model. Instead, name branding in this way risks enacting rigid barriers related to the position.

Regardless of the legitimacy and name branding afforded by this law, other participants described negative impacts that the ACA had within their communities. Juana and Carmen described how, prior to the implementation of the ACA, their local hospital ran a volunteer clinic for anyone who was uninsured. The clinic saw various uninsured individuals including rural White and Black populations in addition to undocumented immigrants. This volunteer clinic provided a variety of services and was either free of charge or on a sliding fee scale. Services included being able to get lab work done for free and see a specialist for as low as $20. As such, this clinic served as one of the few places in which undocumented immigrants could receive (and afford) health care in this community. However, Juana and Carmen informed me, once the ACA and the Healthy Indiana Plan 2.0 (Indiana's term for the Medicaid expansion, known by its acronym "HIP 2.0") went into effect, many of the poor White and Black patients at the clinic were able to acquire some form of insurance and stopped attending this clinic. Due to the lack of demand, the clinic closed despite the need in the undocumented immigrant community. Fortunately, a core group of volunteer medical professionals has continued providing care to the undocumented population in this area.

Challenges in Care: HIPAA, HIP 2.0, and Other Laws

There were additional federal and state laws that created barriers and enacted boundaries for CHWs in the provision of care that also complicated their caregiving. The Health Insurance Portability and Accountability Act (HIPAA) was a landmark federal law passed in 1996 that introduced a variety of policies and practices regarding the collection and flow of patient information to protect against theft and fraud in addition to addressing a variety of several other related issues. HIPAA has predominantly impacted CHWs through their need to learn a variety of forms and practice confidentiality and privacy regarding client information.

While participants understood the value of the law, many found it to be a boundary that impeded their ability to provide care. Laura, a CHW, who works predominantly with Latinx families, described how HIPAA guidelines complicate the provision of care. She explained that, for the Latinx families she serves, privacy laws do not mesh well—as the entire family is often involved in caregiving and discussing medical concerns. While HIPAA is focused on the patient-provider (and ancillary staff) dynamic, for the clients of CHWs, the family unit is an important aspect in the provision of care. Similarly, Carmen complained that she seems to spend more time reviewing HIPAA privacy procedures and guidelines with her clients than time spent engaging with the medical provider. She described her frustrations to me, "They are obsessed with covering their butt legally. There is more time spent on HIPAA than with the doctor. I have no problem with HIPAA being important but that's driving everything now." Thus, while this federal law is fulfilling its imperative to protect the privacy of patients, it also enacts barriers that complicate the provision of care by CHWs to those most in need.

While participants described the barriers enacted by HIPAA, other participants drew inspiration from this law in strengthening their approach to care—and thereby, remaining in the guidelines put forth by this law. The certification course underscores the importance of CHW-client privacy and confidentiality in addition to HIPAA and other relevant policies. Aside from learning about HIPAA, confidentiality, and other relevant policies, students are also taught skills related to observation and listening—emphasized as a metaphor of having "big ears, big eyes, and a small mouth." Essentially, CHWs must be observant, protect clients through their adherence to guidelines, and in the practice of care. These topics were reflected during the photovoice project as well. Isabella took a photograph of a sign at a local hospital that reminds staff to keep patient information private (see figure 4.1).

In her photograph, Isabella coalesces the impacts of law, privacy policies, confidentiality, and her observational training as a CHW. She explained how hearing the client and maintaining confidentiality are two of the most critical aspects within the CHW-client relationship. She explained, "So, I don't have to say much. I just need to be there, I have to be present, and I have to be a good listener . . . but always keeping in mind to keep that discussion private unless it needs to be discussed with the boss lady [laughter]." In interactions with clients, she explained that she practices having big ears, big eyes, and a small mouth to provide a space of trust and privacy—per the guidelines established by HIPAA. Thus, despite participants who voiced frustration related to HIPAA and confidentiality policies, others drew upon them as a source of inspiration and as a reinforcement of their training.

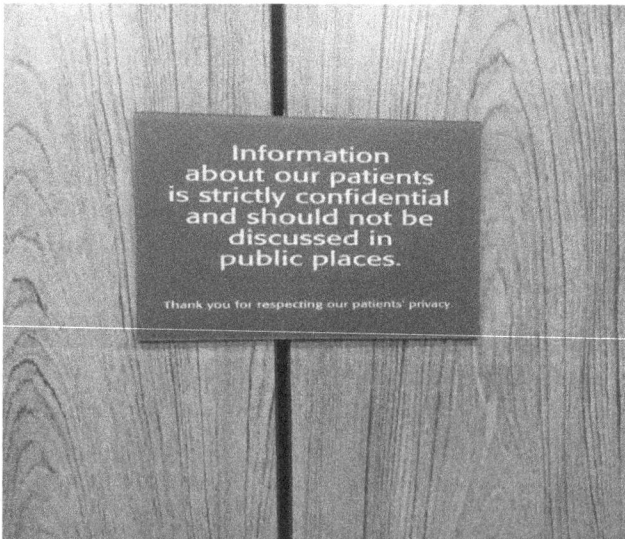

Figure 4.1 "Must have big ears, big eyes, and a very, very small mouth." *Source:* Photo by Isabella (Pseudonym).

Intimately connected with the ACA included the Medicaid expansion offered to states for their governments to opt-in. Indiana was one of the few conservative states that expanded this program, resulting in the creation of HIP 2.0. This program was built from the framework of the Healthy Indiana Plan originally launched in 2008. The plan itself allows for individuals who qualify as a resident of the state as well as falling into specified, federally set income guidelines. Negotiated in 2015 between Indiana and the federal government, federal funds are used to pay for individuals between 100 and 138 percent of the federal poverty guidelines.[5] The program reduced rates of uninsured in the state and, as of December 2017, 397,000 beneficiaries were enrolled in this program.[6]

However, this program has been critiqued as punitive since it penalizes those who are most in need of accessing insurance. HIP 2.0 requires that beneficiaries contribute a portion of their income monthly in order to access this insurance and maybe disenrolled from the program for up to six months for failing to pay the premium within 60 days.[7] While providing many within Indiana to access health insurance, other barriers remained for those who are outside of poverty guidelines or are not residents (i.e., undocumented immigrants). For others though, the fact that they must contribute monthly incomes creates barriers[8] in addition to the fact that individuals who are disenrolled for failure to pay the premium must wait the full lockout period before reenrolling.[9]

The barriers enacted by HIP 2.0 were glaringly evident in the years following its enactment. Rudowitz et al.[10] reported that the two major reasons for who either never enrolled in the program or disenrolled were due to affordability and confusion about the payment process. Participants described issues in helping clients sign up for HIP 2.0 as well as having clients dropped from the program. Andrés explained that he had clients who had been repeatedly disenrolled but had been told they could reapply. However, he asserted that reapplying for the program was needlessly complicated, resulting in a significant barrier for him to help clients as well as serving to discourage clients from attempting to reenroll. Andrés also expressed his skepticism of a repeal of the ACA (and its resultant effect on the HIP 2.0 plan[11]) but did fear the implications that could arise for his clients.

There were other federal, state, and local programs that were, at times, inaccessible for clients of CHWs. "On My Way to Pre-K"[12] is a state-funded program that provides grants to four-year-old children from low-income families in order to help them access high-quality preschools. Carla, a CHW who works within the Latinx community in southern Indiana, described how the state had recently changed the program to require that children of enrollees be the U.S. citizens. She described her frustration with this change while helping a family, "I think it was two months ago, this family was here applying for asylum for Venezuela and it's like they can't join this because they're not citizens and to me that's B.S. because it's not fair to the kid, I mean they're just looking for a better life and you're saying that they can't go to this program because they're not citizens?"

Carla also described the barriers faced by immigrant clients when attempting to access federal and state insurance programs and other benefits. Her clients who had become legal permanent residents had to wait at least five years prior to qualifying for programs such as Medicare, Medicaid, and Children's Health Insurance Program (CHIP). She elaborated,

> Even with insurance you have people who are permanent residents here that have to wait five years to get any type of insurance, they are just limited to emergency services unless they make a certain amount of money then they can apply for the (ACA) marketplace and even so it's expensive, it's not affordable, and it's not fair for those people who are fighting and went through the process of citizenship. For them have to wait that long to get health care, that's another thing that makes it difficult for a lot of my families.

Thus, issues related to immigration status and socioeconomic class are prevalent social determinants of health complicating access to care and resources. These are further exacerbated by government requirements and regulations, denying the deservingness and medical citizenship of the clients served by CHWs. Alternatively, Bob complained that government regulations and policies that are set up to help individuals sometimes create situations that do not help clients that much. He described a story experienced by one of his clients who received benefits from the Supplemental Nutrition Assistance Program (SNAP) (which provides funds to buy foods, commonly known as food stamps). "You talk to them or ask them, 'Ok, well how much in food stamps do you get?'" 'I get $5.95 a month.' What?! What?! What is six bucks in food gonna do you?! But because of the [government] formulas that's all they can qualify for."

While the benefits provided by SNAP are to help enrollees access food, the actual translation of this care at the ground level demonstrates the essential uselessness for this recipient. In attempting to diminish the social determinants of health faced by those in need, the program does little in terms of helping some enrollees. Thereby, CHWs play a crucial role in addressing the need to find additional resources for those facing food insecurity. Ultimately, these laws, policies, and government programs enact complications in the provision of care and provoke unintended consequences that CHWs must negotiate in their caregiving.

ESTABLISHING BOUNDARIES
THROUGH SCOPE OF CARE

The work performed by CHWs varies greatly and is dependent on each employer and/or organization. The set of regulatory guidelines for the roles and responsibilities by which CHWs must adhere themselves to is referred to as "scope of care." This scope is not only mitigated by employer, organization, and specialty trainings but also impacted by federal and state laws. Scope of care was also emphasized throughout the certification course and outlined basic guidelines for this workforce that could be adapted to specific employer designations. Also known as scope of practice, which Berthold,[13] drawing on a Federation of State Medical Boards 2005 report, defines as,

> The rules, the regulations, and the boundaries within which a fully qualified practitioner with substantial and appropriate training, knowledge, and experience may practice in a defined field. Such practice is also governed by requirements for continuing education and professional accountability.

Although there is a wide range of activities and roles fulfilled by CHWs, there is always a scope of care within which they must remain. The scope of care covered in the CHW certification course is broad with the emphasis that this scope of care (in addition to the certification itself) is a foundational training and that the employer must further define the appropriate scope of care. In terms of the certification course, scope of care includes providing culturally competent health education, informal counseling, case management services and referrals, community organizing, advocacy, and recruiting and supporting clients in accessing services. The training repeatedly emphasized that CHWs must remain in their scope of care at all times and to also recognize when and if they feel they might go out of their scope. Scope of care is also protection for the CHW, so that they know how to establish boundaries to protect them from burnout and promote their self-care (topics discussed further in chapter 6).

I asked participants to describe how they determined when to stay in scope, and if they ever felt the need to go outside of said scope in order to help their clients. A common issue I heard from participants is that their scope of care was too broad, leading to trouble in establishing healthy boundaries to maintain with clients and leaving some participants feeling overworked. Part of this issue stems from the fact that the CHW position itself is somewhat vague as there are many roles and responsibilities fulfilled by these workers, which is at once a strength and a weakness.

Andrés voiced his concerns when it came to scope of care, though he had mentioned going outside his scope of care (as mentioned previously by providing his personal phone number to clients), he opined for further refinement of the CHW position. He told me, "Well, as a community health worker . . . I know it's a very broad job description—but I think it has to be, hopefully in the future, a little more defined. I know the people talk about community health worker *pero* [but] we don't have a specific definition, task, a model." He acknowledged during the development portion of this position in Indiana that "I know this is still in the building process but it will be nice to have a really defined description as a community health worker because sometimes, believe it or not, we have to have some boundaries. . . . Otherwise, we'll be so overwhelmed that we won't be able to function."

Andrés went on to explain that instead of expanding his role as a CHW, further definition of the boundaries related to his current responsibilities would better help him in his work. He also argued that further defining the scope of care would be more appealing to potential CHW employers. Andrés asserted "that [establishing more boundaries] would really help to . . . define what a community health worker [is] and it would be easy to present to hospitals and organizations exactly . . . what are their specific tasks and what are also the boundaries they have established." As such, Andrés demonstrates how providing additional framework to the CHW scope of care would help establish boundaries to make the position more appealing to those working as a CHW as well as to potential employers who will better grasp the position. Due to the relative gray area in which CHWs operate, participants described how the ambiguity found in their scope of care challenged them to stay within, or go outside of the scope of care.

GOING OUTSIDE THE SCOPE OF CARE

As described in the opening of this chapter, some participants described facing challenging situations that pushed them to go outside their designated scope of care. For some, it was due to the deep relationship fostered with clients, in which some participants felt more as friends rather than CHW and client. Patricia, a Black woman and a CHW with 24 years of experience, explained that she has had to "restrain herself" at times in order to not overstep her boundaries. She told me, "It's hard because it becomes personal and I don't want it to become personal in the advice that I give. I have to refrain . . . even with smoking it's like, 'Why can't you just stop smoking? We have all these tools.' So, you have to put the brakes on and I try not to cross those boundaries." Patricia had to actively remind herself to remain within her scope of care even if this meant allowing the client to continue smoking—and thus (1) respected client autonomy and (2) remained in her scope of care as a CHW. These boundaries outlined in her scope of care helped her maintain a professional relationship with the client.

For many clients of CHWs, transportation was a perpetual social determinant of health that hampered their ability to access care, food, job opportunities, and more.[14] As a result of the poor mass transit system, many participants described feeling pressured to provide transportation themselves for their clients to and from appointments and to procure needed resources. The majority of participants were technically unable to provide transportation due to not having liability insurance provided by their employer. For some participants, this boundary had to be crossed, especially when policy changes introduced further pressure to do so.

Other participants, who had been cross-trained as CHWs, explained how they integrated their CHW training with their full-time job in order to cross boundaries in their caregiving. Frank, a White man in his early 50s, who is an executive director of a community-based organization, and cross-trained as a CHW and probation officer, described how the CHW training aided him in broadening his view regarding criminal justice. While he previously had worked as a probation officer, the certification course helped him to see how structural factors, such as the social determinants of health, impacted his clients in a myriad of ways that also complicated their probation. As such, Frank was more empathetic toward his clients and provided additional resources and guidance to help them succeed. Many of the cross-trained paramedic CHWs described how the training aided them in being able to focus on the broader environment in which their client lived within, rather than just focusing on the specific injury of the client. The CHW training helped these individuals provide referrals and other resources to prevent clients from having the same issues in the future and thereby prevented further emergency calls. For individuals who maintained employment in a different job, the CHW model served as an additional repertoire from which they could draw on to address the well-being of their clients where they might be pushed out of their scope of care depending on their job.

In spite of the scope of care provided in the CHW certification course and additional employer-designated guidelines, several participants described still going outside of these boundaries. In the majority of these cases, the participants described feeling as though they did in fact *have* to go outside their scope in order to effectively provide care to their clients. As such, laws, policies, scope of care, and negative consequences did not serve as impassable boundaries that prevent some CHWs from doing all that was necessary to positively improve the well-being of their clients. Connecting back to their moral obligation and commitment, these participants justified going outside their designated scope of care in order to help those in need.

CHWs were keenly aware of the significant implications that could arise as a result of going outside the scope of care. While some, such as Carmen's example in the beginning of this chapter, found ways to morally justify doing so, others considered these challenges as insurmountable ethical dilemmas. Thus, reinforcing the decision to stay within the designated scope of care. Making the decision to go outside or within the scope of care was a deeply personal choice, weighed after much thought. It provoked an intense conversation within the minds of these workers, especially as they sought to reconcile their boundaries with ensuring the highest level of care for clients. Martha described needing to do the "right thing" in such cases, when I asked if she ever felt as though she had to go outside her scope of care. She explained,

> I don't feel that I *have* to go out of my scope and personally I always look at it ethically. Am I doing the right thing? It's a decision to stay within that scope, there's no "you *have* to go out of scope,"—you do the right thing. It's an ethical dilemma but to do your job effectively you have to stay in that scope because if you divert for one challenge, then the next challenge what do you do? Then the scope is totally distorted because you did not stay in that scope. Your ethics are distorted and that impacts the scope if you go out of it. Then the scope becomes a non-scope because you're making exceptions here and there and the guidelines lose its effectiveness.

Her description echoed Beverly's thoughts in chapter 2 about whether or not she would help a client who wants to do something that goes against her morals. Thus underscoring the need to understand how moral obligation and value to clients shape the caregiving of these workers.

In order to not warp the scope of care, some participants offered advice and ideas for other CHWs when confronted with situations that pushed them to cross boundaries. Leticia explained her previous work in which she trained registered nurses as CHWs. She told me that in these classes, she emphasizes to nurses that if, for example, they are working in the role of a CHW then they are *not* to fulfill the role of a nurse, including refraining from using their clinical skills. Leticia offered another example of a certified community health worker (CCHW) who is also trained as a medical interpreter. In this case, she asserted that the individual's primary role is that of a medical interpreter, and thus they must serve the role and align with the scope of care of that position. Not mixing these two roles was crucial not only to maintain the scope of care but also to not push the individual to be faced with an ethical dilemma. Juana, a *promotora* who manages *promotora*-trained medical interpreters in south central Indiana, explained,

I have to remind my *promotora* that when you're doing something, I know that you want to help the world, I know you want to solve that problem at the moment but when you're here [interpreting in the hospital] this is what you are going to do. "Oh yes, I can think of this person needs this, this, and this," but when I am interpreting for the doctor, I am not their social worker or anything. You give your card at the end and say "If you need help, I do this [*promotora* work], call me." But just to have parameters and a scope of work.

Several participants were adamant that—regardless of the situation—it was imperative that one must always remain within the designated scope of care. In my conversation with Martha, she described at times struggling to remain within the scope of care but that she never felt as though she had stepped outside it:

No. Sometimes personally, not myself, but as others you want to help individuals but you *have* to stay in your scope of practice. That's not a negotiable because as a CHW no matter what we feel personally we have to stay within that scope because there are those individuals you want to help in ways that might divert out of the scope but the bottom line is staying in that scope . . . I was challenged by this and I saw a person that was in need of something and I thought "should I do this or should I not" because our hearts say we want to help but sometimes we have to bypass that. I think it is fairness if you don't do it for one and then you don't have to decide what do in each and every situation. It's heart wrenching because you want to help but if you make an exception here then what do you do the next time?

Martha demonstrates how being flexible in terms of going out of scope may make one susceptible to completely warping their boundaries for every situation. However, for participants who felt they had to or at least were willing to go out of the scope of care is indicative of the structural violence encountered by their clients. While a scope of care is provided to CHWs and cross-trained individuals, sometimes going outside the scope was justified via a moral standpoint. Ultimately, the broader political economic context that places clients in structurally vulnerable positions directly affects the moral conviction of the CHW in making their decision to stay within or go outside the scope of care.

Issues regarding staying within the scope of care are connected to the broader ambiguity of the CHW model itself. The flexibility of the CHW model comes as both a strength and a weakness as the roles and responsibilities can be adjusted and adapted to the specific needs of the employer and client base. However, this same flexibility comes at a cost in that ambiguity regarding scope of care can lead to CHWs feeling overwhelmed in their responsibilities, which risked experiencing burnout. Given the gray areas encountered by CHWs, maintaining some autonomy will provoke these workers the ability to make their own judgments and calls regarding the provision of care.

COMPLICATIONS OF FUNDING

Many of the participants have boundaries and regulations placed through the ability for employers to fund CHW positions. Indeed, funding has been noted as a "primary barrier" to connect these workers with vulnerable populations.[15] As previously described, many CHW positions in Indiana (and hence the large variation in titles) are due to the fact that these are often funded through short-term grants that last from anywhere between 1 and 3 years and then are dependent on securing additional funding. The majority of health and social services employers may secure a grant but then are unable to secure more funding (or if they are, become stuck in a position of never knowing if they will receive funding the next round). Many of these organizations do not have the financial capital in order to institutionalize the funding for CHW positions. Additionally, these positions may not provide significant pay (and/or benefits) for those working them to consider them as their primary source of income. Thus, enacting boundaries related to the feasibility of these positions (and, again, highlighting their professional structural vulnerability).

Several CHWs related their concerns regarding how tenuous funding, salary, and length of employment negatively affected their well-being. Renata, a CHW who now works for a county-level public health department in Indiana, described the story of how her position transitioned from a soft- to hard-funded position. She told me that the position was only a 2–3 year-funded position and her primary responsibility would be health education regarding lead poisoning within the Latinx community. Although the position was much needed, her employer cautioned her that there was no guarantee of additional funding. Renata, a Latinx woman in her 50s, who was unhappy in her former job, was willing to risk-taking this tenuously funded position. Fortunately for Renata, her supervisor informed her that the health department decided to include her position in "general funding" and thus institutionalized her position. The department also expanded her roles to focus on issues in health broadly and dependent on her community's needs.

While Renata received long-term employment, for many CHWs there is a dearth of well-paid and long-term CHW positions. Miguel, a CHW who had previously worked for a social services organization in southern Indiana, had to leave this very same position shortly after I first met him. When I followed up with Miguel, he had taken a position with a health insurance company because he had better job security, pay, and benefits. Miguel stressed that he still utilizes his CHW training in his interactions with individuals throughout the 19 counties he services. Ximena, who had recently completed her certification, originally took the class as she had been laid off from her job at a health insurance company. However, she was unable to find work as a CHW and eventually found employment with a different insurance company for the same reasons as Miguel—job security, salary, and benefits. Ximena lamented that there are not more organizations in her city hiring CHWs. Instead, she is only able to be a CHW on a volunteer basis. She emphasized that her passion lies with CHW work but the lack of these positions forced her to find work again with an insurance company.

This lack of funding for CHW positions enacts barriers that hinder individuals from (1) being able to find these jobs, and (2) remain in them for substantial time. This creates barriers in fully realizing the potential of these workers and also hinders individuals completely from finding work as a CHW. In spite of the issues detailed in this section, hospitals in large cities including Indianapolis, Fort Wayne, and Evansville began hiring CHWs in the several years. Many of the participants in this study were paid (n = 34) with several additional participants stating they did this work on a paid and volunteer basis (n = 10). Cherrington et al.[16] found that CHWs diverged when compared between a volunteer and paid position. For CHWs who were paid, their obligations aligned with that of the organization while volunteers aligned more with the community.[17] Overall, CHWs are faced with boundaries in pursuing this work. On the one hand, many CHWs in the state are paid for their work (albeit to varying degrees). On the other hand, they face a tenuous situation regarding job security and benefits.

BREAKING BARRIERS THROUGH EVALUATING THE COST-EFFECTIVENESS OF CHW PROGRAMS

In spite of the positive benefits that CHWs can offer within the broader workforce and communities, many employers may be skeptical of CHWs related to the potential for return on investment (ROI) of hiring such workers, thus manifesting as a significant barrier that prevents their employment. Many public health studies have demonstrated the various benefits and positive health outcomes that CHWs can provoke through public health programs or collaboratively with medical professionals. Nevertheless, this still has not led to their broader acceptance throughout much of the United States, especially in Indiana. However, appealing to the potential for cost-effectiveness through instituting CHW programs may be one way to break this barrier. Several studies have demonstrated that CHWs do in fact produce cost-effective out-comes.[18] The sparse number of studies that demonstrate cost-effectiveness (compared to the production of positive health outcomes from CHW pro-grams) is likely indicative of the fact that these workers often exist on the fringes of the healthcare workforce.

Participants in this study were aware of the issue of cost-effectiveness and that it is a missed opportunity. In our interview, Carmen proclaimed, "One thing that concerns me is the lack of value put on the role of the community health worker in saving cost—and cost runs everything!" According to her experience, she not only produces positive health outcomes for her clients, Carmen also reduces spending through her services. She also offered critiques in terms of spending money on apps and other high-tech solutions aimed to remind patients of their appointment yet fail to get to the root of *why* a patient does not (or is unable) attend. Carmen asserted that investing instead in CHWs, these workers would ensure the patient makes the appointments, gets to the pharmacy, gets their medication, understands how to follow the instruc-tions, and the CHWs provide follow-up care. She declared, "That would all be covered if we were part of that [multi-disciplinary healthcare] team," how-ever, she was aware of the potential impact cost-effectiveness might have on her pay, continuing "but again you have to put value on that. . . . 'This com-munity health worker will save us $50,000 a year so we'll pay her $25,000' or whatever. But I constantly see that resistance." Her final words hearken back to chapter 3 in recognizing the structural factors experienced by CHWs in the professional workforce due to gender, race, and ethnicity. While failure to assess cost-effectiveness may prevent CHWs from entering the workforce, there is also the chance that greater cost-effectiveness may negatively impact CHWs pay. Still, she recognized, "We're always missing something for a lack of coordinating care all the way through."

Lucía was also aware of the possibility that assessing the cost-effectiveness and ROI studies on CHWs may remove some barriers blocking their accep-tance into the workforce but offered a nuanced approach for future studies. She asserted that studies should take an economic approach but through analyzing the positive effects CHWs have through keeping the overarching workforce healthy. In expanding on this idea, she asserted that the care CHWs provide creates ripples that extend beyond understanding why a patient is unable to attend an appointment but also impacts work-related issues such as absenteeism and loss of income in terms of not only the individual but also the employer and in tax revenue. Lucía suggests analyzing the ways that CHWs maintain a healthy workforce in addition to how this example may be attractive for companies such as Amazon (specifically for maintaining the health of their warehouse employees) which would have positive financial implications for job opportunities and development in local communities.

The barrier faced by CHWs in terms of their expanded employment within the professional workforce is hampered by their ability to produce cost-effective outcomes along with the production of positive health outcomes. It is possible that this exists but may take years of study to demonstrate cost-effective outcomes following the introduction of a CHW program thus requiring several years of funding before seeing sustained cost-effectiveness in addition to positive health outcomes. Although studies have demonstrated this potential, additional studies should continue assessing the cost-effectiveness of CHW programs. As such, in connection with the previous chapter, their professional citizenship may also be facilitated through their ability to produce cost-effective outcomes. However, as participants noted, additional issues are likely to emerge in terms of reduced salary depending on how much ROI employers can get out of their CHWs. While positive results regarding cost-effectiveness may lead to increased opportunities, it may also have impacts on the position itself as these workers would likely need to produce positive "health" outcomes on the bottom line for their employing organization.

THE ISSUE OF REMUNERATION

Boundaries also emerge for CHWs in terms of their remuneration. A plethora of studies have analyzed issues that emerge between stakeholders, employers, and CHWs related to pay.[19] Many of these studies utilized the framework of moral economy to assess how conflicting views related to pay emerge between organizations and CHWs that exhibited a concern on part of employers that somehow paying CHWs (or increasing their wages) would taint the inherent motivation of these workers. Swartz and Colvin explain how CHWs noted the economic benefits of care work but worried that it would appear "in tension" with the rationale of altruism as the core motivator for care work—thereby describing CHWs as both "carers *and* members of a resource-constrained community."[20] Maes[21] explored the motivations that exist in nongovernmental organizations (NGOs) in Ethiopia for not paying CHWs since they are considered "priceless." In his study, the employers asserted that the "mental satisfaction" of their services should be considered compensation enough for these workers. Maes learned from the well-paid Ethiopian public health officials that CHWs should not be remunerated for their service lest it "'ruin' or 'crowd out' the intrinsic motivations, values, and religious beliefs that underlie CHWs' capacities."[22] Unsurprisingly, the CHWs interviewed by Maes asserted that earning an income would not tarnish their motivation for serving others.

Furthermore, Nading[23] explored the issue of remuneration among CHWs. Workers in this study were "ambivalent" regarding the pay they received in that while it signified their belongingness within the professional workforce, it was also a reminder of their structural vulnerability due to the low pay. Nading also notes that the government of Nicaragua removed a provision that had ensured CHWs receive remuneration, instead reimagining them as "citizen-volunteers" on the part of the government. Other scholars have called for organizations to address the issue of pay. Closser and Jooma[24] assert that these workers must be paid livable wages. I also explored this topic in my studies given the barriers that are put in place through either not paying or barely paying a livable wage.

During interviews, I asked participants about their feelings on being paid versus unpaid in addition to whether or not their approach to care would change. I allowed each participant to answer then briefly explained the various studies carried out by Maes, Closser, and Nading and the background information on how this issue has developed around the world. A significant portion of the participants (61%, n = 30) candidly expressed that being paid would not change their approach and, actually, being unpaid would create a barrier to engaging in this line of work entirely. Participants were also ada-mant that being paid and/or being paid more would not change their approach nor corrupt their motivation for participating in this work. Frank posited, "I don't think you're going to pay people enough in this business to dis-incen-tivize them." Building on this notion, Andrés asserted,

> To be honest, from my point of view I would say that yes, you need to be paid in order to survive. But it's not like a main thing for me, because you have to have that desire. You have to have in yourself the desire to work with people, you know, it's something innate that you like to help people but of course I got the opportunity through this organization to be paid for that, which I enjoy the payment, but at the same time it's kind of equally enjoyment—not just for get-ting paid for that job but it also really rewards me on a personal level that I really feel comfortable and very open to help people no matter what.

Many participants were clear that it is vital for employers to pay CHWs a livable wage and to also understand that their work is difficult. The majority of participants described how, to be a CHW, an individual has to truly be motivated to do this work since remuneration alone will not be a sufficient factor in causing someone to lose (or instill) a moral conviction and motiva-tion for conducting this work. As described in chapter 1, many participants noted that having compassion is the basic requirement and that the technical skills of a CHW can be taught to anyone. Jim, a health program director and manager of two CHWs, told me, "If you get the heart and the compassion and the desire to work in their heart first, you can shape the rest. But you've got to have that foundation to begin with. Of course, if you pay them, they're going to stick around, they can't stick around if they're not going to feed their families." Thus, for the majority of participants, possessing an inherent drive to be a CHW was crucial but that pay itself was just as necessary in order to work in this position as their career.

For CHWs in the United States, participants noted that earning a livable wage was foundational in establishing themselves. While participants noted that pay was an important factor, possessing the inherent drive was equally as essential. The key argument against the NGOs and other employers in the anthropological studies is refuted in these claims by participants—the initial drive is vital to being a CHW but that remuneration will not corrupt their motivation. For some participants, earning more money would increase their motivation and deepen their obligation to their work. Carmen elaborated, "And like anything else your volunteers that are totally unpaid have the free-dom to say 'I can't make it, I can't do this, I can't do that,' if you have an important health fair—[the volunteer may say] 'we're going to be on vaca-tion, I'll be with my grandchildren,' whatever, so that paid position you're going to get more of a response—*an obligation.*"

For CHWs and program directors alike, providing a livable salary was a key component of the position. For participants who had experienced being paid little, it could actually result in a negative outcome in their work. Bianca, a CHW who had worked in positions in which she received low pay, stated, "Being paid a stipend was helpful, but not enough. It did change how I approached my work. From the beginning, I was aware I was not doing the work for the money. However, sometimes it was discouraging to earn so little, it made me feel like my work . . . was not really valued or considered a priority."

Remuneration itself could serve as a barrier, or at the very least a bound-ary, for participants. In spite of claims by NGOs and employers as noted by studies conducted in the developing world that paying these workers would somehow shift their intrinsic motivation, CHWs in the developing world and in the United States asserted it would not. Paying these workers (and offering greater remuneration) would in fact provoke a deeper sense of commitment and obligation, removing boundaries, and, ideally, leading to healthier communities. Carmen further explicated that pay in and of itself is a sign of respect, she described a conversation related to the pay that she and her coworkers had received "...about our salaries, which were pitiful. One of my peers said to me 'you know, your salary is a sign of the respect they have for you.' That slap in the face has never left me." In response to paid versus unpaid CHW labor, she added "You lose a lot when you don't have a paid employee . . . that respect factor is huge." Remuneration is a major factor for making CHW work feasible, desirable, and to remove barri-ers for CHWs. As the government of Indiana professionalizes these workers (and for any other states and countries), it is essential that they be viewed as legitimate health actors providing a distinct service and adequately compensated as such.

CHWS AND THE FRAMING OF BOUNDARIES, BARRIERS, AND CAREGIVING

CHWs encounter a variety of barriers and boundaries in the provision of care dictated by laws, policies, scope of care, funding, and remuneration. Laws and policies that set out to protect patients and/or offer options for health insurance can also complicate the caregiving of CHWs. Laws such as HIPAA that provide protection for patients in terms of their medical history also complicated the provision of care provided by CHWs. Similarly, laws such as the ACA and connected health insurance programs such as HIP 2.0 provide insurance options to many of the clients serviced by CHWs. However, these programs also come with a variety of caveats that also serve as barriers and boundaries in accessing care and resources.

The certification course and employers both provide scopes of care for CHWs. These establish guidelines and enact boundaries related to the practices and responsibilities of CHWs. However, many participants described feeling constrained by these boundaries. For some, the lack of rigidity and flexibility of the scope could be overwhelming. For others, the political economic environment and structural vulnerability of their clients pushed them to go outside of their scope of care to provide services and resources. As such, some participants provided services that potentially had positive health outcomes for their clients but could also result in negative consequences. For these participants, they justified their actions via moral obligation to community and client. This concept is echoed in Buch's[25] analysis of at-home caregivers. These individuals sacrificed their personal comfort in addition to sometimes going outside of the boundaries of their scope of care in order to provide the needed care to clients. The issues surrounding scope of care may be one of coaching and experience—especially allowing more experienced CHWs to coach other CHWs in addressing the various issues they may encounter and how to best remain in their designated scope of care.

Funding and remuneration were additional factors that enacted boundaries in establishing CHW positions and providing their feasibility. Despite studies that have assessed the apparent issues regarding the payment of CHWs throughout the world, participants were adamant that payment and increased remuneration will not negatively impact their motivation to participate in this work, echoing the sentiments of CHWs in Ethiopia and Pakistan.[26] Like their counterparts in Pakistan, CHWs in the United States also need their job to provide a livelihood for them and their families. Thus, similar issues abound in the United States as well reflecting issues in the moral economy of care in both countries.

The following chapter delves into perhaps the most unique role of these workers—advocacy. This role, in particular, has the potential to address a plethora of health issues that often result from social determinants of health. Through this role, CHWs to surpass boundaries that other healthcare providers do not engage in the provision of care. However, steps that professionalize these workers risk reducing their ability to participate in this role—potentially complicating this role and the future of the profession.

NOTES

1. Backe 2018; Brodwin 2011; Buch 2013, 2014; Closser 2015; Nading 2013; Stevenson 2014.
2. Garfield et al. 2019.
3. Bovbjerg et al. 2013, Katzen and Morgan 2014.
4. In Indiana, the Medicaid expansion is known as the "Healthy Indiana Plan 2.0" (HIP 2.0).
5. Semuels 2016.
6. Rudowitz et al. 2018.
7. Goodnough 2020, Rudowitz et al. 2018.
8. Semuels 2016.
9. Rudowitz et al. 2018.
10. Ibid.
11. For more information on the implications of a repeal of the ACA and its effects on the Medicaid expansion, see https://www.kff.org/policy-watch/eliminating-the -aca-what-could-it-mean-for-medicaid-expansion/.
12. For more information, see https://www.in.gov/fssa/carefinder/4932.htm?utm _source=google&utm_medium=cpc&utm_campaign=2020-enrollment&utm_con- tent=0.
13. Berthold 2016: 34.
14. Logan 2020.
15. Schmit et al. 2021.
16. Cherrington et al. 2010.
17. Ibid.
18. See, e.g., e.g., Allen et al. 2014, Brown et al. 2012, Cross-Barnet et al. 2018, Fedder et al. 2003, Gaziano et al. 2014, Mirambeau et al. 2013, Vaughan et al. 2015.
19. Closser 2015; Maes 2015, 2017; Maes and Shifferaw 2016; Maes et al. 2014, 2015; Nading 2013, 2014; Swartz 2013; Swartz and Colvin 2015; Takasugi and Lee 2012.
20. Swartz and Colvin 2015: 140.
21. Maes 2015.
22. Ibid.: 108.

23. Nading 2013, 2014.
24. Closser and Jooma 2013.
25. Buch 2013.
26. Closser 2015, Maes 2012.

Chapter 5

"So That No One Can Belittle Them"
Advocacy as Caregiving

Advocacy is a defining role of the CHW model and a unique contribution they offer to the health and social services workforce.[1] Advocacy can take many forms, including calling utility companies (to get an extension on a bill or to not cut off services for clients), asking that medical professionals clarify diagnoses, helping clients find solutions to barriers (due to social determinants of health), and engaging with politicians to affect policy change. While some of these activities may not seem strictly related to health and well-being, they are pivotal to addressing the many needs of clients and community *outside* the clinic that directly affect their ability to improve their lives.

Perhaps the best way to illustrate the various ways in which CHWs engage this role is captured by my time spent shadowing Andrés. While the majority of Andrés's clients are immigrants from Latin America, he has also established himself within other burgeoning immigrant groups in his town including those from the Marshall Islands and Moldova. Embedding himself within these various groups is essential in order to help each navigate potential social determinants of health that may affect these communities differently as a result of their structural vulnerability. Andrés told me, "And when I go to advocate with somebody, I'm really into it. Like if I see somebody that doesn't have a way to get that [resource] or to have their voice listened to in the community, I'm that voice for them. I advocate in any situation: it could be a legal situation, in a school situation, a personal situation, et cetera."

His participation in advocacy does not stop on the clock, he also engages in this work in his free time including health education, finding new resources for the various communities, interpreting in both medical and legal situations, and translating forms into Spanish. He also participates in community organizing (another role of CHWs intimately connected with advocacy) within the Latinx community regarding issues such as health, community safety, and planning cultural festivals. Andrés emphasized, "This is one of my other passion areas—that I advocate for them to help them . . . feel safe, *verdad* [right]? To make them see that they can trust somebody to go along with them to solve or try to solve the problem they might encounter." As such, Andrés draws on his moral obligation and commitment to his community while also drawing on the trusting relationship he maintains with his clients in the moral economy of care.

As previously described, Andrés was unique in that his official title is "community health worker" but also serves as a medical interpreter. During the time I spent shadowing Andrés, he was tasked with interpreting during several appointments in the morning hours and then shifted into conducting several hours of community outreach. Andrés was also in a unique position as he was provided use of a car owned by the clinic, thus he could transport clients as designated by his scope of care due to possessing liability insurance from his employer. As we drove throughout the town, Andrés demonstrated his extensive knowledge of the community, describing his connections with local churches, food pantries, and Latinx grocery stores. We also discussed advocacy and the primary role it serves in CHW's work. Andrés recounted a story to me in which an unscrupulous organization was charging immigrants as much as $300 to fill out an individual taxpayer identification form—in spite of this being a freely available form. He related this information to the Latinx community coalition, of which he is a member, and the coalition developed a program to aid immigrants in completing their taxes and providing any necessary forms for free.

Andrés drove us around the various neighborhoods in which he serves. At one point, we passed by several used car dealerships, Andrés informed me that he knows the majority of the owners in addition to which ones he recommends to his clients. He bases this information on stories from individuals in his community and other business owners, ones who had learned the hard way after being ripped off by some of these car dealers. Andrés connected the provision of this knowledge to his clients to advocacy, as finances are a vital resource for immigrants and he wants to protect their resources from being taken advantage of.

During the final part of our day together, Andrés interpreted for a monolingual Latinx man who was meeting with a lawyer. Andrés client had been injured on the job and was running into barriers as he was trying to access workers' compensation. In contrast to his counterparts that are required to serve simply as a mouthpiece (unless they wanted to go outside of scope), Andrés would occasionally interject questions to the lawyer to clarify specific points, such as what kind of documentation and information is required so that there would be no confusion later. Following the appointment, Andrés clarified that if he thought of a certain question to ask the lawyer, he would first ask his client—asserting that the question must first be asked by the client before he would translate it to the lawyer. In this form of advocacy, Andrés highlights how he engenders empowerment—suggesting the question but leaving it up to the client's autonomy to ultimately decide if it should be asked.

Throughout my time spent with Andrés, he addressed a variety of issues at different levels. From advocating for individual clients at medical and legal appointments, in health education, and through community outreach and as a member of the Latinx community coalition. Andrés actively works to improve not only the individual lives of his clients but also the broader community in which he lives. Many other CHWs also participated in this wide range of advocacy in order to circumvent the deleterious impacts of structural violence and improve the overall well-being of their communities. The centrality of advocacy was a prominent theme that emerged through other aspects of the study. Camila, a CHW who worked for a large hospital in Indianapolis, posed a photograph and caption (see figure 5.1).

For Camila, being a CHW was equivalent to advocacy—and advocating for anyone in need regardless of race, ethnicity, nationality, or socioeconomic

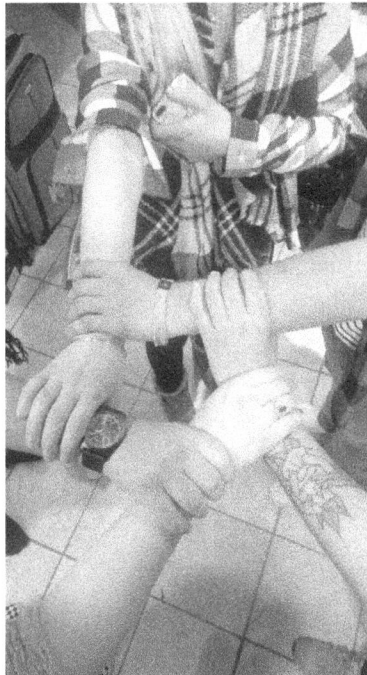

Figure 5.1   "For me, being a CHW means advocating for others no matter their skin color, religion, economic status, or nationality." *Source:* Photo by Camila (Pseudonym).

status. In this chapter, I delineate advocacy along with three primary "levels of impact" as well as assess the challenges CHWs faced while advocating. In doing so, I demonstrate how CHWs draw on advocacy to create change for individuals, communities, and the broader society. Given the potential for advocacy to enhance the lives of clients, I assert that advocacy must be considered a form of *caregiving*.[2] The findings I present here contribute to the work of other scholars who have analyzed CHW advocacy and assessed how it shapes these workers, affects clients, and provokes policy change.[3]

ANALYZING THE "LEVELS" OF CHW ADVOCACY

As noted in Andrés's and Camila's examples, advocacy forms the crux of their work as CHWs. I documented CHWs participating in advocacy aimed at creating an impact at three distinct levels, which are comprised of advocacy that occurs at the micro, macro, and professional levels[4] (see figure 5.2). Micro-level advocacy creates impacts for individual clients and provokes changes at the organizational level (e.g., in hospitals, community-based organizations). Macro-level advocacy is aimed at creating impacts within the community and broader society. Professional-level advocacy occurs in the workplace and can be split into two sublevels (1) in which CHWs must advocate other professionals regarding the legitimacy of their position and (2) in which CHWs must advocate their own employer for resources, programs, and other necessities either they or their clients need. At times, there may be some overlap between impact at these distinctions but can largely be split up along these three levels.

Table 5.1 displays examples that participants took part in for each level of advocacy. I argue that parsing out advocacy in this way provides simple grouping structures that demonstrate various activities and roles CHWs partake in to show how advocacy serves as a form of caregiving. These categorizations provide practical means for employers, potential employers, and

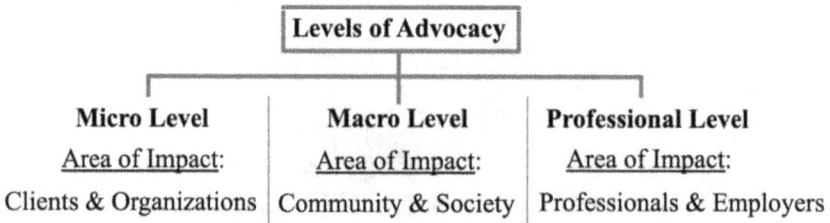

Levels of Advocacy		
Micro Level	**Macro Level**	**Professional Level**
Area of Impact:	Area of Impact:	Area of Impact:
Clients & Organizations	Community & Society	Professionals & Employers

Figure 5.2   Levels of CHW Advocacy and Specific Area of Impact. *Source:* Figure by the Author.

Table 5.1 Examples of CHW Advocacy at Each Level

Micro-level Advocacy	Macro-level Advocacy	Professional-level Advocacy
Changing policy at the hospital, clinic, and/or organizational policy	Attending political rallies and/or demonstrations	Advocating professionals regarding the legitimacy of the CHW position
Standing up on behalf of clients to medical professionals and/ or insurance representatives	Meeting and collaborating with politicians (local, state, federal) to address health and community issues	Advocating employer to not cut funding for community programs and other provided resources
Providing health education and engendering empowerment	Participating in community mobilizing to address issues or plan events	Speaking with professionals, potential employers, and policy-makers to spread awareness of the CHW model
Finding and connecting clients to resources and following up	Encouraging clients to attend town halls to meet with political representatives about issues	CHWs organizing for better wages or rights in their work

medical professionals to view this kind of work to improve health outcomes and well-being.

ADVOCACY AT THE MICRO LEVEL

While CHW participation in advocacy differed between the three various levels, all participants took part in advocacy at the micro level. The majority of participants described their participation in advocacy generally through educating and engendering empowerment within their clients—this directly connects the act of empowerment as an example of micro-level advocacy. Health education becomes a form of advocacy, according to participants, because clients, for example, may be unaware how to care for themselves, may not fully comprehend their diagnosis and treatment plan, and/ or may be unsure how to overcome social determinants of health that bar them from accessing care. Other common forms of micro-level advocacy described by participants included follow-up (in order to ensure referrals and resources helped clients) and continued support in connecting clients to resources.

Many participants leveraged their connections within the community. Andrés negotiated resources for clients such as deals on cars, appliances, and other resources. Participants also advocated at the micro level through signing clients up for insurance, educating qualifying clients of insurance benefits, contacting utility companies to not shut off clients' electricity, water, and/ or gas in addition to helping clients purchase minutes for their cellphones. Veronica, a cross-trained paramedic and a CHW, once helped a client attain a free, new furnace from a local community organization in Indianapolis after her client's old furnace had died in the winter. Although the examples discussed so far tend to demonstrate how CHWs provide services and resources to clients, many participants emphasized that engendering empowerment was an essential component of advocacy. The provision of these resources, they asserted, must be provided in a way that illustrates how clients can learn to navigate the economy for resources and/or speak up for their own needs.

Micro-level advocacy also occurred when clients advocated to change hospital, clinic, or organizational policies in order to better facilitate individual client care and needs. Various examples of how participants advocated at the micro level included having hospital, clinics, and social service organizations put up signs in multiple languages to direct patients and clients to proper locations to access services and getting hospitals and organizations to include forms in multiple languages. In several cases, participants themselves had to either translate the forms or find copies online. Additionally, for CHWs who worked within the Latinx community and other marginalized populations, participants served as a trustworthy source of information and access to the healthcare system. Camila explained how she tells immigrant clients where they can access care and resources in addition to letting them know that they will not be reported to Immigration and Customs Enforcement (ICE) if they seek care. Similarly, Rosa told me that much of her advocacy is related to informing clients regarding how to access resources. She engenders empowerment by having them take the first step in asking for said resources and encourages them to access them, lest they disappear if the need is not manifested.

Advocacy at the micro level could also blend into having larger, community-level impacts. Gabriela explained how she advocated for hospitals to be aware of cultural differences in patient populations and to specifically provide signs in Spanish to help her individual clients navigate the healthcare system. She explained,

And then the other way [of advocating] is making sure that organizations are aware of cultural nuances that will alter the way that services are rendered to the community. So, I advocate while not for an individual patient, I advocate for the people group by bringing up questions and finding out. If there is a hospital in Johnson County that doesn't have any signage in Spanish, advocating for our people that there needs to be signage in Spanish so they know where to go get their services.

Gabriela notes that instead of advocating for one person, she seeks to change the experience of her entire community through her actions. In doing so, Gabriela changed the way the hospital approached accessibility by getting them to place signage in Spanish to better help her client and future Spanish-speaking clients.

One of the most common forms of micro-level advocacy described by participants was speaking up on behalf of clients. This was an important role for CHWs as it helped patients cross a communication barrier—as they could lack confidence in speaking up for themselves or felt powerless in the medical professional-patient relationship. Many times, CHWs described speaking up as asking for clarifications regarding diagnosis, prognosis, and/or treatment plan between a client and medical professional. Others stated they had spoken up for a client if they felt their client was being condescended to or discriminated against. However, most of the time this action was done in order to clarify diagnosis or at least speak in simpler terms to help clients better understand a procedure. Gabriela explained how even with an interpreter, clients may still be unsure of what is happening; underscoring how providing understanding is a form of advocacy provided by CHWs:

Patients don't usually understand what really is happening to them and what their care plan is, even though they have an interpreter they really don't understand it because they [the interpreter] don't explain "What does this *mean?*" I mean they [the interpreter] may tell them, "You're going to have a cath[eter]," and they use terminology that is too high and, so helping them understand [is a means of advocating]. And they use numbers like, "Your risk number is 9." Well, 9 out of what? So, advocating for them is making sure that they understand what their treatment plan is and understand what is really happening to them. That helps them end up knowing what . . . they [the patient] need to do differently to comply. So, that is one way of advocating.

Gabriela elaborated, noting how advocating for clients includes ensuring that the "right" questions are asked, especially in regards to how the social determinants of health may deleteriously affect their ability to carry out a treatment plan or address chronic health issues.

The other way is making sure that the right questions are asked. They [the patient] may be too nervous to [have the medical professional] find out, "Ok, [I don't have] transportation, I don't have enough food, I need to pick between insulin and this other expense." So, helping ask the right questions even though they haven't thought about it. I will always do that for the patients so to me all of that is one way [of advocating].

While CHWs took the lead in standing up for clients or asking the right questions, they asserted that including clients in these interactions (such as on a phone call) and coaching them on how to do this themselves was vital. Rosa and Valeria were both adamant that while they are a resource and advocate for the client, the client should make the call and take the lead. However, they asserted that following up with the client was essential to make sure the need was met and, if not, they would take the necessary action to acquire the resources or services needed.

Participants who were Affordable Care Act (ACA) navigators would help walk clients through signing up for insurance best suited for each client. Again, the process was used as a teaching mechanism for clients to see how to navigate the market but have an expert who could instruct and advocate for them throughout the process. This concept of aiding clients through the convoluted U.S. healthcare system was a ubiquitous theme among CHWs. This theme also appeared in the photovoice project. Gabriela responded to the prompt, "What is an impact you have had as a CHW?" by showing a photograph and the accompanying caption (see Figure 5.3).

Her photograph displays an individual standing at the banks of a powerful river. Just as many of her counterparts described their advocacy simply as

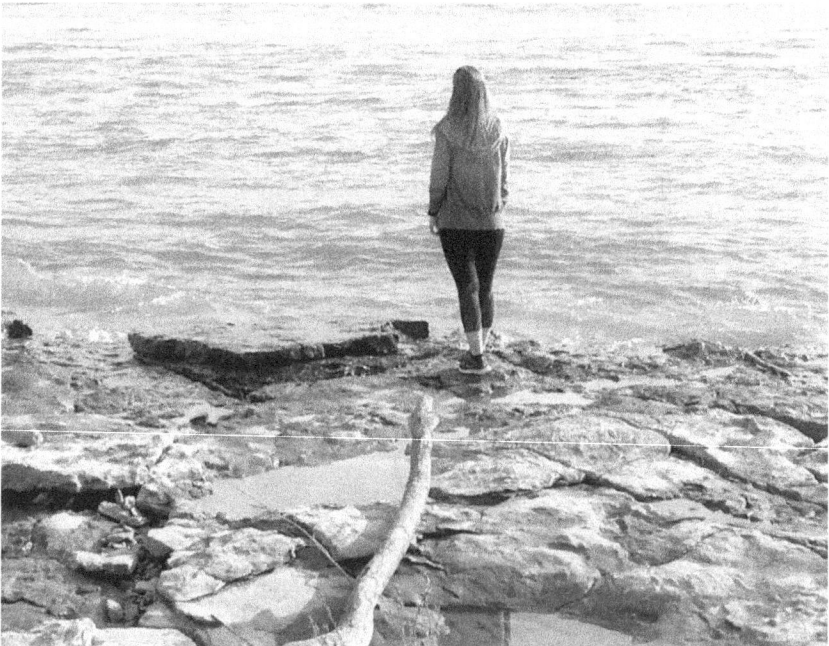

Figure 5.3 **"Helping patients know how to jump into the health care system."** *Source:* Photo by Gabriela (Pseudonym).

providing access to health care, Gabriela described her impact as a CHW as helping clients navigate the healthcare system. She expounded that the river in the photograph serves as a metaphor for the U.S. healthcare system—one that is intimidating for people to cross and for many, if they attempt to forge it, become overwhelmed by the current of its complexity. Thus, demonstrating how the U.S. healthcare system itself is impassable for many. As a CHW, however, she serves as an advocate for her clients by helping them navigate the river of the U.S. healthcare system and connecting them with other resources and services to best suit their needs.

Engendering empowerment was an outcome expected by CHWs at this level of advocacy and was demonstrated when clients advocated for themselves in the various situations where the CHW had taken the lead. As established in chapter 2, participants asserted that their work should not result in perpetually holding the hand of the client but serving to unlock self-confidence and self-sufficiency through engendering empowerment; with empowerment being achieved over time through their service and advocacy. Maricela explained her approach in aiding clients with the caveat that they attempt to help themselves, "So when a client feels that they need advocacy, what I can do is I say 'How can I help you help yourself? It would be great if you did it yourself but if I can help you do it, yes.' So I always ask that question, 'How can I help you help yourself?'" In this way, CHWs draw on their connection to clients, trusting relationships, and advocacy within the moral economy of care to positively affect the health and well-being of clients.

Aside from engendering empowerment, one CHW described that her biggest form of advocacy is validating her clients' feelings. Vanessa, a cross-trained CHW and paramedic, asserted, "You have a PhD in you." Vanessa explicated that this validation was a crucial component to engendering empowerment in addition to other forms of micro-level advocacy. She argued that this led to additional self-confidence in medical and social services appointments and thereby instilled belief in the individual regarding their own self-confidence. In this way, the CHW served to engender that confidence through validation and help clients overcome this barrier in taking control of their own lives.

Advocacy at the micro level produces outcomes that aid clients and serve as one contribution CHWs offer within the professional workforce. These various examples illustrate the diverse ways participants helped their clients surpass barriers and boundaries in accessing resources and health care and circumvented the social determinants of health. Participants also demonstrated how advocacy at this level is essential in engendering empowerment and self-sufficiency. This is due in part to the direct connection the CHW facilitates with the client and the individual strategies developed to address any struggles experienced by the client. While empowerment remained the ultimate goal, participants emphasized that they will always be a support for their clients—even for those who become empowered.

ADVOCACY AT THE MACRO LEVEL

Macro-level advocacy consisted of a variety of activities that were aimed at creating impacts within the community or broader society largely through participating in community coalitions, attending political demonstrations, mobilizing the community to address issues of concern, encouraging clients to attend town halls and write to their representatives, and engaging directly with local, state, and federal politicians. Macro-level advocacy did not have to be explicitly political, other CHWs participated in organizing health fairs and cultural festivals that could connect the community and positively affect social, mental, and physical health. Participating in advocacy at the macro level could sway change in the form of law and policy to affect community health and, thereby, lead to health equity. However, this form of advocacy was more divisive for participants, with fewer participating in activities related to macro-level advocacy.

Unlike its counterpart at the micro level, macro-level advocacy was almost always done while not at work. This was due in part to the fact that often macro-level advocacy could blur into political activism. Several participants took part in community coalitions that sought to address issues within the city. Beverly volunteers her time as a member of such a coalition in a large city in northern Indiana with a significant Black population. A large part of her time, she told me, is advocating for the needs of the Black community. She asserted that many of these needs are available in other parts of the city but are inaccessible for her clients and broader community. In her participation in this community coalition, she explained that she does not feel her opinion is always welcomed. Beverly stated,

> There are just things that should be happening on the south side of town that are not happening. And so I am on a coalition that is fighting for things to be happening on that so I'm a little bit aggressive on that portion of it. I'm the only person of color on that whole coalition. And sometimes I'm sure that I'm not well received [laughter].

I remarked how it sounds as though she's unfazed by this poor reception and remains resilient in her advocacy for her community. Beverly replied, "I am [unfazed], I am advocating for things that need to happen over here. We [speaking on behalf of her south side community] don't really care about a bike trail, not as much as a grocery store and a safe place for kids to be, a playground . . . so I don't really care about a bike trail. I don't really care. I care about it down the line but this is what this community needs [now]."

Thus, regardless of the poor reception Beverly receives, she still participates in macro-level advocacy in order to secure the needs of her community as a whole. Her persistence is vital to improve the social well-being of those in her community with change being attained through the passage of municipal policies that enact change in communities that are most structurally vulnerable in comparison to other populations of the city. Additionally, Beverly's participation in this coalition is underscored by the fact that she does so during her free time, typically after having put in a full day's (or full week's) work. Aside from demonstrating her commitment to her community, this again highlights the unpaid labor completed by CHWs advocating for change at the macro level.

Several other participants were members of committees, collaborations, or coalitions that sought to improve the well-being and social health of a neighborhood, community, or minority group through networking, planning events, and connecting to resources. Activities carried out by these groups included reaching out to local, state, or federal politicians or lobbying to pass a measure or policy to address issues in the community such as food deserts, safety/crime, and/or public transportation. Some CHWs encouraged their clients to write letters, attend town halls, or go to the offices of their elected officials to inform or inquire about issues or changes. Patricia told me that when community issues arose, she would pose the question to her clients, "Who has the power?" to remind and emphasize that *they* have the power and tools to provoke change.

Aside from serving on community organizations, other participants directly organized their community members and clients concerning political issues. Marcia, a CHW and director of a health organization in a large city, is involved in a variety of macro-level advocacy activities. She regularly calls local legislators regarding issues in the community. She also invites these legislators to town halls she organizes on a quarterly basis to discuss issues occurring in her community. When organizing these town halls, Marcia passes on this information to two of her employed CHWs as they do outreach to people affected by the problem as potential community members who can speak on the issues to the legislators. Some of the issues Marcia has been involved in trying to inform legislation on includes public transportation, potable water, infant mortality, and health translation. Other participants engaged in the political process by writing letters to their representatives in support of the Deferred Action for Childhood Arrivals program (DACA) and meeting with politicians in person to express their support for the ACA and its Medicaid expansion in Indiana (i.e., the "Healthy Indiana Plan 2.0 [HIP 2.0]). Some participants attended political demonstrations to stop the deportations of undocumented immigrants from an airport outside of Gary, Indiana.

Macro-level advocacy also occurred outside of the political realm. Several participants attended local chamber of commerce meetings or were members of neighborhood committees that planned events to bring communities together (such as a Latinx heritage festival). Some participants participated in an apolitical form of macro-level advocacy that also effortlessly blended advocacy at the micro level. Miguel, a CHW of Puerto Rican descent, participated in several fundraising events aimed at providing resources to Puerto Rico following the destructive wake of Hurricane Maria in 2017. While this action can be considered a form of macro-level advocacy, he also performed micro-level advocacy through working to bring 30 families from the island to Indiana and helping each of them locate jobs and other resources.

These examples illustrate how advocacy at the macro level can generate impacts for the broader community and society, and thereby, improve the well-being of many. At times advocacy at this level could blur into political topics such as protesting in support of DACA, the ACA, and against deportations. Additionally, encouraging clients to attend town halls and engage with local, state, and federal politicians sought to empower clients to become more involved in issues in their community and at the national level. However, other times participants took part in organizing health fairs and cultural events that were apolitical yet produced positive social and physical health outcomes at the broader scale.

ADVOCACY AT THE PROFESSIONAL LEVEL

Finally, CHWs participated in advocacy at the professional level. This advocacy particularly highlights the barriers CHWs encountered in their work environment. As noted earlier, professional-level advocacy can be split along two distinctions: (1) in which CHWs must advocate for the legitimacy, awareness, and dignity of their position to professionals, stakeholders, legislators, potential employers, and the public; and (2) in which CHWs must advocate to their employer to expand the provision of resources or to not cut programs that promote the well-being of clients and community. The latter is similar to advocacy at the micro-level, however, in this case, CHWs were advocating directly to their employing organization rather than an outside organization or clinic. Previous scholarship has assessed CHWs advocacy directly to their employing organization and/or in forming a union to protest for better rights and wages.[5]

As noted in chapter 3, CHWs who worked as medical interpreters described how, at times, they would go out of scope in order to provide care for patients, which can be considered a form of micro-level advocacy. These CHWs also advocated at the professional level by advocating doctors and medical staff to increase the availability of medical interpreters. Likewise, as noted in chapter 4, many of these CHWs felt restricted in their scope of care when they were stuck to translating and were forbidden to advocate or discuss other issues. However, some participants, such as Carmen, stepped out of her scope as an interpreter and sought to advocate for the patient while also informing the doctor of her ability to fulfill other services. In this way, these participants advocated directly to the medical doctor (and staff) to expand their roles as interpreters and thus integrate more of their roles as CHWs within the clinical encounter.

Outside of the medical realm, in social services and community-based organizations, CHWs also participated in professional-level advocacy. In these cases, participants described advocating to their employer to better foster social justice for their clients and broader communities. Patricia told me how the Black community in her city had encountered discrimination when seeking help within her organization:

> I also advocate for them—the family health center in the community did not have a diverse staff and a lot of folks in public housing felt they were being mistreated in that center. I shared that with the director during our board meeting, "This is what I'm hearing in the community." It didn't happen overnight but she made some changes. She wound up hiring a Black receptionist and spoke with her staff. That is me advocating for my community and that organization made changes and now they didn't have to wait three months to be seen.

In Patricia's case, advocating at the professional level during the board meeting and informing her employing organization about the discrimination experienced by her community members helped to provoke systemic change that translated to better experiences for her clients and community. Additionally, Patricia's example demonstrates how CHWs can fuse advocacy at all three levels: (1) at the individual level through addressing issues of discrimination that affected the individual, (2) at the professional level by advocating her board of directors about this negative experience, and (3) at the macro level through institutional changes to better facilitate services provided to the community. This underscores how advocacy can occur at multiple levels and institute changes to better affect the provision of services, foster a culture of inclusivity in the organization, and foster the well-being of the wider community.

CHWs working in these organizations have encountered significant barriers in their professional work life and have had to advocate their employers to find additional sources of funding and/or not cut specific programs benefitting their communities—including CHW programs. Valeria explained that she was initially hired to work as part of a grant-funded, pilot position. Her position was eventually moved to institutionalized funding and she now advocates to her employer to hire at least one CHW at their other seven branches. Marcellus, a Black man in his early 60s with seven years of experience as a CHW, told me how he experienced homelessness and substance use disorders following his time in the U.S. military. He described how he has advocated for his own position and the importance of continuing financial support for CHW programs:

> I advocate for my job as a CHW every day. Because I've actually in the past gone to bat with my employer for them to continue the work of community health workers or to continue a community health worker program. And just advocating and telling them about the value and why we should fund it and why we should try to find that funding. And if we discontinue it today, can we bring it back tomorrow? Because I'm always advocating for the community it's not just about the program itself. It's basically every time the community loses a program it's a disadvantage but if they have to lose a community health worker program, it's double the disadvantage.

Marcellus' comments highlight the issues brought up in the previous chapter, underscoring the need to institutionalize funding streams for CHWs and related programs. Alisha also has advocated to her employer for a larger role in the process of implementing CHW programs. She's also repeatedly explained the perks that employing additional CHWs could bring in an organization—connecting to economic arguments in asserted "community health workers are the return on investment, *we* are the ROI." As noted in the previous chapter, the few cost-effectiveness studies have shown positive results for CHW programs, and, perhaps combining it with advocacy at the professional level could help institutionalize CHW funding and result in additional CHWs being hired.

CHWs also had to advocate to their employers regarding their own self-care needs. A primary concern of participants was the lack of a unified hub for CHWs in which they could get help, speak with other CHWs, compile available resources, among other potential uses. Isabella argued that addressing and advocating among CHWs and their employers for self-care is important to preserve the health of these workers. She stated,

> We need talk about how a community health worker does self-care and advocate for themselves and how they're still being able to help others but also keeping themselves mentally stable and healthy and having a good mental state. That's one of the hardest things to do because I see it for myself personally as

a community health worker. I want to go out and help my community but when I myself am feeling down and overwhelmed, who's going to help me? Where do I go, what do I have to do? That's something we need to talk about and we need to share with each other what Alejandra [a CHW] is doing to help herself or what Carmen [another CHW] is doing so that way we can help each other and uplift each other.

In my discussion with Leticia, she reiterated Isabella's points and added that CHWs need an internal advocate since they are the "new kid on the block" in the professional workforce. Leticia also asserted that CHWs will need to continue to be their own advocate since they will likely experience pushback from other professionals as they continue to enter the workforce. These comments describe two connected issues: the need to participate in professional-level advocacy for oneself and experiencing stress on the job that can lead to burnout and compassion fatigue; especially if self-care is not prioritized by the employer.

I also asked participants whether they had felt as though they had to advocate for the legitimacy of their own job. Several participants, particularly for those who worked under a title different from "community health worker," described not having encountered this issue. In connection to chapter 3, this is likely due to the fact that under this different title (especially for medical interpreters) they possessed professional citizenship in which other professionals viewed them as a legitimate presence in the clinical encounter. Other participants, especially among those not employed in a clinic or hospital, would accompany a client to a doctor's appointment and would use the term "patient advocate" in order to gain a passing sense of professional citizenship. While this served as a means to gain fleeting professional citizenship and removed the need to advocate, it failed to spread awareness of the position. Mike, a White man in his 20s and a CHW, described his frustration due to this lack of awareness stating, "If we didn't have to explain what we were doing every time we talk to someone first, it would be easier."

As described previously, several participants who had been long-time CHWs were now predominantly working behind the scenes on the certification class. Their primary responsibilities included working on the professionalization of the model, meeting with potential employers, and spreading awareness. The latter two activities were of vital importance to advocating, professionally, regarding the CHW model. When I asked Martha if she has had to advocate for her own job as a CHW, she explained, "My personal job, no, but speaking for our workers what we are going through now working with WorkOne [a workforce development agency] and being able to speak up and advocate for the benefit of having community health workers in the health arena." Illustrating how a primary role is to advocate for the broader acceptance and hirability of CHWs. She continued, "That is somewhat challenging because a lot of health organizations don't know what community health workers can do. For example, we have a good relationship with Meals on Wheels, but they're saying, 'We serve meals, what do we need a community health worker for?' . . . that person gets a meal, but are they eating it? Is it conducive to what they want? Some people have food but they don't want to eat alone. You know? So, they [the community-based organization] miss that social part."

Martha explicated, "So, being able to advocate not for my job but for the job of those who actually are out there because I'm more on the training side. However, interjecting into that, being able to help others see the values of community health workers and getting on the medical teams so that individuals don't have to come back to the hospital. . . . So, I have to take the other side on that—I haven't personally had to fight for my job as a community health worker but supporting all the workers that we do have out there and seeing what challenges they have."

She elaborated how she is interested in developing a marketing campaign aimed at spreading awareness of CHWs throughout the state as another means of professional advocacy for this workforce and, thereby, further building the professional citizenship of these workers. Martha's work is another example of CHWs participating in professional-level advocacy—underscored by her advocating for the utility of the position as well as for its broader awareness and acceptance. As noted by Leticia and Martha, as CHWs continue to become integrated throughout the state, advocacy for their professional needs and legitimacy will be vital to facilitate this transition and, thereby, provide another legitimizing mechanism that could foster professional citizenship for these workers.

Similarly, I attended three of the CHW task force meetings and personally witnessed Lucía advocate at the professional level for the position. In particular, she interjected crucial arguments and material regarding the need to consider the impact of the social determinants of health, maintaining the advocacy component of the model, asserting for the benefits of certification, and recognizing that CHWs must serve as coresearchers in research projects. She also advocated against the overmedicalization of the position and noted that many CHWs do (and should) work for social service agencies and that these CHWs not be forgotten. Lucía also would clarify how certain changes to the core competencies and other policy issues may serve to hinder membership within this workforce in terms of its accessibility.

Overall, many participants described having to advocate not only for their client and/or broader community but also for their own position. This professional-level advocacy encompassed their advocacy for the legitimacy of their position and/or for their professional needs. This level of advocacy demonstrates how these workers are active agents in their professional needs in addition to underscoring how this type of agency can become tiring and lead to burnout and the need for self-care. While all participants interviewed in this project participated within at least one of the levels of advocacy (if not all, at some point), there were a variety of challenges that emerged at each of these levels.

CHALLENGES IN ADVOCACY

While advocacy is a core pillar of the CHW model, there were challenges unique to each level of advocacy in addition to some that cut across all levels. For some participants, macro-level advocacy could be a barrier for those who did not want to participate in activism or take on political causes. These participants felt as though advocacy at the broader scale was not for them, choosing instead to focus on the smaller scale and push for change at the micro level. Others were unable to participate in macro-level advocacy due to employer restrictions, at least while on the clock. Although these participants sometimes took part in macro-level advocacy, such as helping to organize a cultural festival or other community event, and instead, tried to remain apolitical in their intent. Andrés told me,

> I'm not trying to be political [laughter]. But if it's something that can be done at the political level without too much involvement, I might be able to be part of it—but I'm not trying to be involved in any political parties. My main concern is to advocate to those politicians to see how can they improve some areas that need improvement or to create new areas of health for those individuals in our community.

While Andrés may engage with politicians, his primary goal is to work with anyone who is willing to change the health landscape and foster positive change. Other CHWs, such as Valeria, also eschewed macro-level advocacy that bordered too closely to politics. She told me, "I try to steer clear of political agendas. Only because I see myself as a community advocate for good. I don't want to be seen as I'm on this side or on that side. I try to keep myself neutral." Valeria elaborated that she also wants to be seen as neutral among her clients so that they may more readily identify with her. For several CHWs, participating in macro-level advocacy was either too much for them to undertake, especially attending political demonstrations or taking a side that might jeopardize their ability to build connections and relationships with clients.

Other participants described the challenges they faced when advocating at the macro level or when engaging a group of stakeholders. Frank, a CHW and probation officer, described his frustrations when collaborating with various actors, especially when the overarching system, as he described, is "broken." He asserted how this, as a result, can lead to disillusionment with macro-level advocacy. Gabriela echoed Frank's sentiments and told me how participating in advocacy at the macro-level can be a double-edged sword, one that can motivate but also demoralize, stating, "It's [participating in advocacy] a double-edged sword [laughter]. So, it does motivate me to do the right thing, I mean it gets me excited when it works. But it's also I know that sometimes a policy change is like climbing Mount Everest without any gear. So, you know that this is a tall one, so it's going to be hard. So it can, on my bad days, discourage me very much but then on my good days my stubbornness kicks in and I'm going to do it. [laughter]. So, it's both."

She expounded on her earlier response and compared advocacy at the micro level to the macro level, explaining how she visualizes where she wants her client to be and uses this abstraction to motivate her approach to caregiving, "And in an individual level, when you are advocating, you see your patient and you see a patient that is healthy even though they have kidney failure and they have all of these things, you see a patient that could be very healthy that could do just a little bit of things [to become that healthy patient]. So, you are advocating for an imaginary patient because you are advocating for what they *can* be rather than what they currently *are*. So, that micro-advocacy has a lot of rewards because if you can get them to glimpse at that person that you're seeing, then the change comes." However, Gabriela noted that the advocacy at the macro level is especially difficult and even more so if the CHW is working on behalf of a marginalized population. She explained, "But advocacy at a greater level I would say is more discouraging than encouraging, particularly for a [marginalized] group that is not well liked."

Aside from the challenges in terms of disillusionment and demoralization that can be provoked through participation in macro-level advocacy, other participants stated they did not have time to take part in this type of advocacy. Patricia told me that she wished she could participate more in advocacy that could affect her broader community but that she is already overcommitted with work obligations. Carmen reiterated similar issues but does try to participate in activism off and on.

Other participants took part in politically engaged, macro-level advocacy albeit on a more casual approach. These participants would be willing to sign online petitions or send pre-written scripts to politicians for a cause they or their community supports. As such, the CHW could "advocate" by showing their support without having to become too personally engaged in the political process. One CHW told me that while she does not participate in macro-level advocacy, she does encourage her clients to speak to their political representatives and informs them of town halls and other means to connect with political leaders. Thus, in spite of some reticence, inability, or unwillingness to participate in advocacy at the macro level, many participants still engaged in this type of advocacy in order to foster change within the broader community and society.

While the majority of participants engaged in micro- and professional-level forms of advocacy, there were still challenges in these levels. This was especially the case when clients were seemingly disinterested in becoming empowered or did not meet expectations in attaining self-sufficiency. Frank explained how this is a challenge at the micro level:

> There is an old saying, "if you're doing for people what they can do for themselves, then that's enabling. But if you're doing for them what they can't do for themselves, that's actually helping them." . . . But if I'm working way harder than they are . . . and they're just like "whatever" then or if my expectations for people are way up here and they can't meet those or even if they're down here [my expectations] . . . it's hard . . . so, you want to advocate for people but you also got to know your limits. And that's a hard thing, it's a hard call.

Many CHWs attempt to engender empowerment through micro-level advocacy but could encounter barriers set in place by their clients. However, Frank's example, which was echoed by other participants, demonstrates when it may be necessary for the CHW to step back. Not stepping back could cause the CHW to experience burnout as they continue to help a client who does not seem to want to become empowered. Participants still emphasized advocating and aiding these clients with any challenges or health concerns.

There were also challenges present when advocating at the professional level. As Isabella noted, there is a lack of a central hub for CHWs in which they can find support. For participants who work as a medical interpreter, they are technically unable to advocate for the client or for an expansion of their role (i.e., integrating more of their CHW repertoire). Although some participants still spoke out about these issues, CHWs still lack professional citizenship; making their need to participate in this level of advocacy necessary but also strenuous and thereby negatively impacting their mental well-being. For others, there was a worry their employers would not secure additional funding or possibly cut programs desperately needed within their communities.

In spite of the challenges found within the various levels of advocacy, this role is a fundamental pillar of the CHW model. Through advocacy, CHWs circumvent challenges and barriers to health and well-being that the biomedical approach fails to address. Although the CHWs in this study did not always conduct advocacy in each of the three levels, all participated in micro-level advocacy to positively affect the health of individual clients. Advocacy must be viewed as a form of caregiving that provides CHWs with the means to help individuals and communities make salubrious advancements toward well-being and health equity.

ADVOCACY AS CAREGIVING

The various examples highlighted in this chapter have documented how CHWs participate in advocacy with individual clients, organizations, communities, the broader society, and within their profession. Regardless of the specific level of impact, the CHWs in this sample demonstrate how advocacy is embedded within the position and functions as a form of caregiving.[6] Advocacy as caregiving is underscored through circumventing the social determinants of health and making care more accessible and more just for clients.

Advocacy can generate positive health and social outcomes and address systemic issues related to racism, discrimination, and structural violence. These populations face various layers of structural vulnerability that is further exacerbated by gender identity, sex, sexual orientation, race, and ethnicity. Many of these populations are seen as "undeserving" of care and/or as "noncompliant." The political climate during the research was overshadowed by the Trump administration attacks on immigrants and communities of color—through rhetoric against their deservingness to care, attempting to repeal the ACA,[7] and attempts to cut funding to programs such as Children's Health Insurance Plan (CHIP),[8] Supplemental Nutrition Assistance Program (SNAP),[9] and Medicaid.[10] CHWs work with clients to develop strategies to address these issues while at the same time advocating to—and, quite often, educating—doctors, organizations, policy-makers, and other stakeholders about these issues. In advocating at the macro level, CHWs defend programs at risk of being cut, stand up for their communities publicly, and push for change at the policy level.

However, due to their lack of professional citizenship, participants were tasked with having to advocate on a professional level. Advocacy as a form of caregiving is still present in this level—highlighted through CHWs advocating for the retaining of specific community programs that benefit their community. CHWs in this regard uplift the voices of their community members to their employers who may be unaware of how cutting funding for a particular program may deleteriously impact the well-being of the broader community. This was especially true if an employer planned to cut a CHW program as noted by Marcellus that it's a disadvantage to lose a program but it's "double the disadvantage" to lose a CHW program or position. In the case of professional-level advocacy, its vital for (potential) employers to recognize that CHWs, through advocacy, ameliorate (or, at least, lessen) the deleterious impact of the social determinants of health but this is only so long as CHWs are able to advocate and be supported in this form of caregiving. Understanding the forces that shape the moral economy of care (e.g., how policies, rhetoric, and deservingness are interwoven in producing vulnerabilities) is essential in underscoring why CHWs must be permitted to advocate to circumvent the social determinants of health and produce the biggest impacts.

It is precisely within this moral economy of care that CHWs—the majority of whom are from marginalized populations—are motivated to help their communities. This commitment to advocacy and obligation to their communities was prevalent through discussions of advocacy. Gabriela asserted,

> And there's the thing, is that community health workers, because they are from the community, they are from an oppressed people group. Naturally. We are first from an oppressed group. And we are learning to stand up to defend our people and what happens is you come against resistance . . . we need to understand that we have a right [to advocate] and we were one of the oppressed and we do have the voice to speak for all the people behind us.

This need to advocate and stand up for communities was also reflected for CHWs as a workforce. Lucía explained, "How do you put a value on that [advocacy]? And in the training, I think that that came through a little bit. But it's really kind of how do we care for this workforce, how do we take care of the workforce to advocate for them so that no one can belittle them." As such, professional-level advocacy for CHWs is needed to protect themselves and ensure they can continue as advocates for their community.

These examples highlight the shared structural vulnerability between CHW and community in addition to underscoring the moral obligation of the CHW within the moral economy of care. As such, CHWs intimately understand (and have experienced) the impact of structural vulnerability from (and within) the healthcare system as well as shedding light on the professional barriers present in their lives. Other scholars have explored how CHWs are also impacted by the same structural forces as their clients.[11] This sense of shared structural vulnerabilities shapes the nature of CHW obligation to community and motivation for advocacy.

Additionally, structural vulnerability intimately shapes how CHWs participate in advocacy as a form of caregiving within the clinical encounter and when providing resources, referrals, and health education. Alisha drew on her lived experience as a biracial, single mother who had also experienced homelessness as factors that shaped her advocacy and caregiving. She stated, "I can't give the referral for one thing and not ask the right questions to find out what's really wrong? What's *really* wrong? Because it's bigger than just the food issue." Her lived experiences shaped her interactions with this same client—as she uncovered her client was going to have his electricity and gas shut off. Alisha learned that it was these issues that were his priority in his life—not taking his medicine. While doctors would have labeled him as non-compliant, it was structural forces exerting pressure in his life that, in turn, affected whether or not he would take his medicine. Alisha explained how doctors would always tell her "you're always able to get something out of them [the clients] that we can't." It is the shared experiences between Alisha and her client, who exist in the same moral economy and had experienced similar issues that allow her to connect with her client at a deeper level and, as a result, advocate for him to find ways to not have his utilities shut off and educate the medical professionals about these other issues impeding his care.

The political economic context which structures the moral economy of care shapes the interactions and participation in advocacy between CHWs and their clients. Shared lived experience is crucial in these relationships as well as shared background including ethnicity, race, gender and/or shared experience with homelessness, substance use disorder, or mental health disorders. For CHWs, such as Gabriela, she operationalized this shared experience and vulnerability of her community in order to provoke change at the macro, micro, or professional level. Advocacy, as conceived by Gabriela, is not only a core tenet of the position but a "right." Additionally, she asserts that "we [as CHWs] *were* one of the oppressed" but since they are advocates and leaders in their community are now able to speak up for their fellow community members.

However, advocacy as a whole and especially at the macro and professional levels can stand at odds with the professional citizenship of CHWs within the workforce. As a result, this can enact barriers and boundaries which bar the acceptance of CHWs. Engaging in most forms of macro-level advocacy—due to its potential to blend into the political realm—is barred for many while on the clock. As the workforce continues to be professionalized, there is a concern that advocacy may be lost.[12] This is already a potential reality in Indiana given the lack of reimbursement for advocacy, which is indicative of how advocacy is devalued by policy-makers and within the professional workforce. Rosenthal et al. caution "if the CHW role is defined narrowly . . . then the historic role of CHW as change agents who work for social justice could be lost."[13]

Ultimately, advocacy must be conceptualized as a form of caregiving and recognized as a foundational aspect of the CHW model,[14] especially during policy development and steps to professionalize these workers. In understanding the various levels of impact, stakeholders, policy-makers, and (potential) employers can view the ways that advocacy positively affects individual and community health. In this way, CHWs operationalize advocacy as a form of caregiving to improve overall well-being and push for health equity. As such, steps can be taken to ensure that advocacy is not written out of the CHW model as this position is professionalized but rather that this core role is maintained. However, it is vital that—in adopting and recognizing the salubrious impacts of advocacy—CHWs are not seen as shouldering the burden of creating wide-scale systemic change themselves. Colvin and Swartz[15] assert that although CHWs can and do have a part in fostering change, other actors and stakeholders must come together to make wide sweeping changes at the societal and policy level to push toward health equity.

While advocacy can foster a variety of changes, the examples from this chapter demonstrate that it is difficult and can place CHWs in a position of contention. Additionally, as noted throughout the previous chapters, the work of CHWs is often unpredictable, difficult, and complex. Burnout and compassion fatigue were topics that also rose to prominence during my conversations with CHWs—as well as the need to foster and value self-care. In the following chapter, I examine how CHWs experienced burnout and compassion fatigue and the steps they took via self-care to heal from these traumas.

NOTES

1. C3 Project 2018.
2. Logan and Castañeda 2020.
3. Closser 2015; Ingram et al. 2008, 2014; Reinschmidt et al. 2015; Sabo et al. 2013, 2015, 2017; Wiggins et al. 2013.
4. Logan 2019.
5. Closser 2015, Maes 2017, Sabo et al. 2015.
6. Logan and Castañeda 2020.
7. For more information, see https://www.ajmc.com/view/republican-attorneys -general-file-briefs-to-repeal-aca.
8. For more information, see https://www.wsj.com/articles/congress-leery-of -trumps-cuts-to-childrens-health-program-1525822614.
9. For more information, see https://www.cbpp.org/research/food-assistance/ presidents-2021-budget-would-cut-food-assistance-for-millions-and.
10. For more information, see https://www.cbpp.org/research/health/trump-admin- istrations-harmful-changes-to-medicaid.
11. Closser 2015, Nading 2013, Maes 2017.

12. Lehmann and Sanders 2007, Nading 2013, Pérez and Martinez 2008, Rosenthal et al. 2011.

13. Rosenthal et al. 2011: 257-258.

14. Logan and Castañeda 2020.

15. Colvin and Swartz 2015.

Chapter 6

"You Cannot Pour from an Empty Cup"

Burnout, Compassion Fatigue, and Self-Care

"But I, in my opinion, it's impossible not to experience this [burnout and compassion fatigue]. If you're going into the job of a CHW, you should know going into this that you are going to experience burnout and compassion fatigue. It's just the reality of it" Alma, a Latinx woman in her 30s and a CHW who is currently working to train others in the certification courses, told me when I asked if she had ever experienced these deleterious conditions that negatively affect not only the individual experiencing it but also the quality of care. Burnout and compassion fatigue abound at all professional levels in the medical and social services workforce.[1] Alma continued, noting the need to rely on coworkers and healthy coping mechanisms to address these conditions, "having supports for someone within your own colleagues, within other CHWs, like what do they do [to cope with burnout/compassion fatigue]? You know, do they go run? Do they . . . make an activity with their family or something? And something that's outside of a job is also important."

Uncovering and understanding the impact of burnout and compassion fatigue is vital to support this burgeoning workforce and determine the best ways to address these deleterious conditions. Most notably, the CHW certification course emphasizes the importance of self-care. Students were asked to identify what personalized forms of self-care they practice and to find ways to integrate this into their daily (work) lives as a means to decompress and destress. Alma has found ways to combine her forms of self-care into her work as a CHW when aiding clients, particularly for those who have or are dealing with a traumatic event, she told me:

> You know, some clients really don't have much of a relationship with their providers but they have an excellent relationship with their CHW and they confide in them and they talk to them . . . just anything and everything that could

141

possibly be said and done and the comfort level that exists is very important. So, I often also write things down. That's something that I kind of got as a kid where I would do a lot of journaling and you kind of just put all your thoughts in that one thing and just let them stay there and carry on.

CHWs had to be cognizant of the accumulative stress that can occur via hearing and sometimes witnessing traumatic events in the lives of their clients, which takes the form of secondary trauma. This form of trauma is defined as "the transfer and acquisition of negative affective and dysfunctional cognitive states due to prolonged and extended contact with others . . . who have been traumatized."[2] Although Alma asserted that it is all but certain that CHWs will—at some point—experience these deleterious conditions, she described other ways of overcoming these issues via support from colleagues, other CHWs, and loved ones to alleviate the impacts of burnout and compassion fatigue. Finding balance through self-care, according to Alma, was vital to protect mental health, process secondary trauma, and provide the highest level of care to clients. She explained, "Just to keep that balance, as much of a balance as you can have. But, yeah, there's different things that I've tried. Like I said, the journaling one I think has been the most consistent one and other things that's just going through the motions and seeing what feels best at the time." Thus, practicing self-care was vital to balance and diminish the damaging effects of burnout, compassion fatigue, and secondary trauma.

In this chapter, I analyze experiences of burnout and compassion fatigue among CHWs in addition to how they employed various strategies of self-care to ameliorate these conditions. I explore how participants encountered these issues in their work with clients and how, through systems of support, they addressed experiencing these conditions. I assess how caregiving is impacted within the CHW-client relationship as a result of these conditions and, in doing so, underscore the need for employers, potential employers, and policy-makers to ensure that CHWs have support with these issues as they are incorporated in the workforce.

At the end of our conversation, Alma offered some additional positive outlook from experiencing secondary trauma and the need to practice self-care to effectively care for others while also protecting the mental, physical, and emotional well-being of CHWs. She explained:

So, you have to keep going and you have to use these experiences as almost testimonies to . . . encourage others that may be seeking something like this either as a client or as a CHW. Just because we've gone through our fair share of negative experiences, doesn't mean that we can't turn them into [something] positive.

And I know that sounds very idealist and . . . very cliché but . . . oftentimes, it's really what pulls you through. . . . Because again, if you burn out completely, you're not gonna be able to carry on and it's so important to have that motivation and that encouragement to say, "You know what? I'm able to make a difference through this line of work and I have to take care of myself to be able to do that."

BURNOUT AND COMPASSION FATIGUE

Burnout and compassion fatigue[3] are similar yet distinct[4] deleterious conditions, which affect those employed in health care and social services.[5] Burnout, however, can occur in any profession and is defined as "a work-related stress syndrome resulting from chronic exposure to job stress."[6] At any given time, up to one in three physicians experience this condition.[7] Burnout typically has a gradual onset that worsens over time, arising from feelings that a worker's efforts make no difference and is exacerbated by a heavy workload, a non-supportive work environment and/or chronic workplace stress that goes unmanaged.[8] It can manifest as a lack of energy, emotional exhaustion increased mental distance from one's job, feelings of negativity regarding work, a sense of low personal accomplishment, and a reduction in professional efficacy.[9] Left unaddressed, burnout can manifest as physical conditions (e.g., chronic headaches, chronic gastrointestinal problems, chronic physical fatigue) as well as mental health disorders including depression, chronic sadness, and chronic mental fatigue.[10]

Compassion fatigue affects those in health care and social services and is defined as "the negative effects of working in a psychologically distressing environment on a person's ability to feel compassion for others"[11] thereby compromising the ability for caregivers and health workers to function in their full capacity. Specific signs of compassion fatigue include reduced feelings of sympathy or empathy, feelings of dread associated with caring for another (and associated feelings of guilt), feelings of inequity within the caregiver-patient relationship, poor work-life balance, and/or a diminished sense of career fulfillment.[12] Additionally, symptoms can manifest within the mind, body, and social health of the sufferer and include headaches, irritability, anger, or anxiety, insomnia, weight loss, and problems in personal relationships.[13] Anthropological studies have assessed how compassion fatigue and burnout manifest in medical paraprofessionals, which also underscore the need for self-care practices and greater access to treatment for the paraprofessional.[14]

Like any other healthcare professional, participants also suffered from burnout and compassion fatigue. Throughout the project, CHWs described experiencing stress, lack of specific responsibilities, feelings of being overwhelmed, tension with management and/or other health and social services professionals, failure to engender empowerment, and disillusionment with advocacy (at all of the levels of advocacy described in chapter 5). Participants also experienced secondary trauma through hearing and/or witnessing traumatic events of their clients.[15] Even though the CHW is not the survivor of the trauma nor directly experienced it, secondary trauma still accrues within these workers and negatively affects their well-being and ability to provide care.[16] With the stresses of the job and the impact of secondary trauma, CHWs must practice self-care to protect their mental and physical well-being while also ensuring they are able to provide a high level of care.

Self-care has been noted as a protective factor that can prevent and/or reduce burnout and compassion fatigue among medical professionals and paraprofessionals.[17] Other factors such as social environment (i.e., the structure and functioning of the workplace and interactions with coworkers) are key areas to address in reducing and preventing burnout.[18] Although the certification class offers training on when CHWs should remove themselves from stressful situations, how to identify the impact of secondary trauma, and various strategies for practicing self-care, there is still a great risk for CHWs in the state for experiencing burnout and developing compassion fatigue. As such, CHWs must have institutional support for practicing and having employers value self-care in order to ensure these workers remain physically and mentally capable of conducting this work.

The following sections explore the ways CHWs encountered situations that provoked stress, burnout, and the strategies participants developed to assuage these issues.

"I'VE NEGLECTED TO TAKE CARE OF MYSELF": EXPERIENCES WITH BURNOUT AND COMPASSION FATIGUE

Given their place in the moral economy of care, the political economic context, structural violence, and navigating care for client and community, CHWs are impacted at all sides by stressful situations that can compromise caregiving. A variety of factors contributed to participants experiencing compassion fatigue and burnout. Much of these issues at the workplace connect back to chapter 4, regarding scope of care and employer guidelines related to the responsibilities of the CHW employees. Lack of defined scope of care, job ambiguity, and exposure to stress have previously been documented as causes for burnout in CHWs and their counterparts throughout the world.[19] Unsurprisingly, research has also demonstrated that stress and burnout are important predictors of job satisfaction among CHWs.[20] However, at the time of writing, research on burnout and compassion fatigue among CHWs in the United States. appears to be minimal. As such, reporting on experiences related to burnout and compassion fatigue in addition to strategies of self-care are essential, especially as these workers are increasingly incorporated into the professional workforce.

As Alma noted earlier in the opening vignette, she and other participants felt as though experiencing burnout was an inevitability of the job. Previous examples which provoked burnout have been discussed throughout the book, including situations in which participants left their phone on after work hours and/or providing personal cell phone number to always be available to clients "just in case" in spite of employer guidelines against this practice. This practice, which sought to solidify the relationship between the CHW and client in the moral economy of care, produced obligations on the part of the CHW that incurred deleterious effects on their mental and physical well-being. Other participants took part in volunteer activities that were often aimed at supporting their community through community events, town halls, engaging with politicians, participating in health fairs, and other events. As described in previous chapters, this constitutes unpaid labor that CHWs partake in. Although their participation within these events was voluntary in nature, they still could provoke stress on part of the CHW since they had to commit their time and energy into these activities. As such, their participation in these volunteer events could also serve as contributing factors to experiencing burnout and/or compassion fatigue.

In the summer of 2019, I traveled to the Community Health Workers' Organization of Indiana (CHWOI) to conduct follow-up interviews with several participants. I specifically asked about their issues with burnout and compassion fatigue. In my follow-up conversations with Isabella, I asked her about her experiences with compassion fatigue and she told me, "Oh, yeah. Most definitely. I think that I've had mental breakdowns. I've had . . . even a spiritual kind of breakdown . . . I'm so exhausted. And because I've neglected to take care of myself because I'm always worried about all my clients that I've neglected to stop and take care of myself." She noted that this particularly occurs when she does not hold herself to maintaining "healthy boundaries" in her work as a CHW. She expounded, "But that's something that I've learned now is that I need to have those healthy boundaries. And I need to set some time aside for myself. So, I've learned to do that. I've learned to, you know, just kind of analyze the situation and see, okay, do they really need me or they're just being extra. And that way, I kind of protect myself too." Isabella continued, poignantly describing how she was brought to these mental breakdowns due to how she had originally approached her caregiving and how she has since shifted her approach:

> But I think that I've learned because before I think maybe a few years ago, I was just like, I don't care what I have to stop doing to go rescue them. I would stop what I was doing [to help them] . . . Now, thinking back, how wrong I was because I wasn't educating them. I wasn't teaching them to be self-sufficient to be empowered to do it themselves because they always had me. And I always came to the rescue. So, I was handicapping them, instead of teaching them.

Other participants also noted the need to develop "healthy boundaries" to serve as a protective factor from experiencing compassion fatigue and burnout. Having an attitude toward their clients of "rescuing them" was seen as erroneous rather participants noted the need to get back to the basics of educating and engendering empowerment. By providing the tools, health education, informal counseling, and instruction, with the goal of having the client eventually taking self control. Thus, these boundaries served to protect the mental health of CHWs, especially from some clients' reticence to take the lead in their own healthcare needs. Similarly, enacting limits and drawing boundaries by hospice care workers and nurses (ideally) served to protect their health and diminish the effects of burnout and/or compassion fatigue.[21] However, as described Lo and Nguyen, "these acts of boundary-drawing became moral dilemmas between self-preservation and the mission to give back to the community."[22] Many CHWs in this study also experienced this moral dilemma in their pursuit of caregiving.

Many participants felt as though their workday was never truly "done," which could leave them feeling stressed and anxious. Especially noting that CHWs lack professional citizenship within the broader workforce, this directly contributes to the stress experienced as a result. Carmen also spoke to this, asserting that lack of infrastructure was an essential factor that contributes to her experiencing burnout. She described being given medical forms at the last minute that she had to translate on the spot and not being told ahead of time by hospital staff of patients changing appointments, which resulted in her showing up and waiting. She stated, "I [as a CHW] seem to be the last to know. I'm not in the loop. No respect, no clout, you know, that problem." These feelings had built up over time for Carmen and lead her to feel increasingly jaded about her work and, ultimately, contributed to her experiencing burnout.

Vanessa had experienced similar issues in terms of her compassion fatigue being caused by workplace stress. When I spoke with Vanessa, a

White female in her late 20s and cross-trained as a CHW and paramedic, about her experiences with burnout, she explained that she pushed herself very hard due to having "unmeetable goals;" including seeing as many as 18 clients within an 8-hour workday. Vanessa explained, "The numbers were absolutely unattainable. And I just threw myself deeper and deeper and deeper and deeper into it. At the end of my time with [my organization], I had nosebleeds. I had night terrors. I wasn't sleeping. I wasn't eating right. And I finally said, 'I can't do this anymore.'" Vanessa's example highlights the mental and physical manifestations of burnout. After experiencing this, Vanessa left her job choosing instead to work outside of health care for a time.

Beverly explained that she has experienced compassion fatigue and how it can adversely affect her abilities, "It can negatively affect [your work] because you're so tired. You're so burned out and stuff. You do things without even thinking about it sometimes and that can be a negative effect." Beverly went on to describe experiencing tiredness and irritability—noting that the particularly negative impacts it can have on clients. Andrés also told me of his experience with compassion fatigue and how it was exacerbated due to the unpredictability of his work schedule.

Structural violence and the social determinants of health also contribute to burnout and compassion fatigue within this workforce.[23] Leticia explained that CHWs have encountered burnout from being repeatedly unable to access resources to aid clients. Although many resources were typically available to CHWs and their clients, they often came with a variety of strings attached as only some clients qualified for particular resources or certain resources may be only available in certain counties. Thereby highlighting how the political economy of Indiana contributes to CHW burnout. In this case, participants felt stuck as they could not get the resources needed to effectively help their clients.

Additionally, aside from the precarious care that is provided to clients when a caregiver is experiencing burnout, the emotional, physical, and mental well-being of the CHW is directly compromised. This directly highlights the insidious cyclical effects of burnout: the CHW experiences stress, contributes to burnout, provides increasingly less efficacious care and services, becomes physically and/or mentally distant and incapable of carrying out the work, ultimately removing the CHW from providing care and possibly leaving the CHW with lingering, deleterious physical and mental health conditions.[24] For many communities serviced by CHWs, the loss of this worker can cause significant harm to a population in desperate need of services and care. As such, considerations for how external forces such as the political economy, workplace responsibilities, and relationships impact these workers and their caregiving. Taking into account these issues is essential for employers, policy-makers, and other stakeholders to support the CHW workforce.

Although in the minority, several participants asserted they had not experienced burnout or compassion fatigue. Juana, a soft-spoken, middle-aged woman from South America and trained as a *promotora* and CHW, argued that she had never felt as though she is not going to help a client because she is "tired" or "burnt out." While she had complaints or issues related to workplace stress, issues with particular clients, and structural factors, Juana relied on a set of boundaries and scope of care to guide her work. Her impeccable approach to these latter factors instilled a preventative form of self-care that protected her from burnout and compassion fatigue. Despite describing issues related to infrastructure contributing to burnout, Carmen described not experiencing compassion fatigue from her clients, stating, "Actually no, [experiencing compassion fatigue from clients] because I get so much out of it [serving as a CHW]." Carmen relied on her compassion for her clients and her position within the moral economy of care to motivate her through frustrations that she experienced from clients, the workplace, or the broader environment. In this case, the satisfaction she derived from her clients served as a protective factor from experiencing compassion fatigue. Juana's and Carmen's examples highlight how CHWs can draw on their morals and connection to their clients as one form of protection against these deleterious conditions.

Ultimately, CHWs in this sample had a wide range of experiences that arose from burnout and compassion fatigue. The factors that contribute stress to these conditions can largely be lumped into three primary categories: (1) clients, (2) the workplace, and (3) structural factors. In examining and taking into account how these various categories influence and contribute to burnout and compassion fatigue, more profound understandings can be ascertained in learning how to prevent these factors leading to these conditions. Supporting these workers is essential and understanding their challenges and frustrations are key topics that must be practiced by policy-makers, employers, and other stakeholders.[25] In combating burnout and compassion fatigue, CHWs practiced various strategies of self-care.

SYSTEMS OF SUPPORT TO PREVENT (OR REDUCE) BURNOUT AND COMPASSION FATIGUE

Given the variety and breadth of experiences participants had with burnout and compassion fatigue, practicing self-care strategies was essential to prevent or reduce the impact of these deleterious conditions. However, broader institutional, community, and employer support is essential to ensuring CHWs can practice self-care, and, feel supported to do so. Participants identified that this support is needed to help them remain mentally, emotionally, and physically capable of aiding their clients and community. Participants asserted that the broader environment should function as a central source of support for CHWs to help cope with the effects of burnout and compassion fatigue. Juana, in particular, noted the need for this source of support. According to her, CHWs must feel broader support, and, in particular, having the community and the state demonstrate this support is crucial for CHWs and preventing these deleterious conditions. Her assertion speaks to the lack of professional citizenship experienced by CHWs as well as how more buy-in from the government and broader public could serve as an additional legitimizing mechanism. Juana stated that people in the state must realize, "'Ok yes, we *do* need community health workers.'" Having increased recognition, institutional funding, and more resources would help to ease their workplace stress and provide enhanced care to clients while, at the same time, diminishing (and preventing) the negative effects of burnout.

Others also noted how the political economy and structural forces need to be addressed in order to diminish the effects of burnout and compassion fatigue. In particular, participants noted the need for additional resources to be available. As Leticia described in the earlier section, the lack of resources in certain areas or for certain populations can provoke burnout among CHWs. In terms of a system of support, Leticia asserted that funding resources such as transitional housing, food pantries, and support for such populations as the LGBTQ+ community and formerly incarcerated individuals will not only provide aid to those in need but will facilitate the ability for CHWs to function efficaciously and, thereby, prevent the buildup of burnout. This sentiment was also echoed by Martha, who asserted having access to all available resources that CHWs could easily look up and access for their clients would help prevent feelings of burnout. In drawing connections to Juana's argument, Leticia stated "because it can get exhausting when you only have a couple of things you can refer your clients to. And it depends on the community and what the community is capable of providing."

Other participants noted how management can take an active role in supporting CHW needs for self-care and in order to prevent or reduce burnout. Marcia explained that as a manager, she engages with her CHW employees, stating, "Well, I think as an organization, we need to keep in mind that the kind of work that CHWs do, they do become really involved with the individual and with the families and it does impact their lives, and be flexible . . . allow them to adjust their schedule for a day, take them out to lunch, and just talk about what's going on." She added that a question employers can and should be asking, "How can I help, as management?" As such, taking an active role as an employer and directly engaging with the CHW employees is a vital step in serving as a system of support.

Some participants suggested alternative strategies. Marcellus suggested that CHWs work in pairs. In his organization, he works with a fellow CHW and asserted that this can be helpful in stressful situations. If one starts to become overwhelmed or stressed, the other CHW can take over. And, if one of the CHWs needs to go on vacation, it can occur without significant impact in the community since the fellow CHW can take over during this time. Andrés also stressed that although he is the only CHW employed at his clinic, having support from his coworkers is vital to his self-care and feelings of support.

Camila also explained how her employer could help provide a more robust system of support. She stated that, at times, her caseload can be very heavy and stressful due to needing to meet certain employer-dictated quotas. In response to this, she asserted that employers must ensure CHWs can take their mandated morning and afternoon breaks to prevent burnout from occurring. The heavy caseload quota can leave employees feeling as though they need to work through breaks. Beverly also noted how work can become stressful due to a high caseload, stating, "It's loving work because you're helping people. But it can be strenuous work because you have a lot of people that depend on you." Potential and current employers can consider these suggestions as the model is further developed and integrated in Indiana as one strategy to employ to provide support to their employees and prevent burnout from occurring.

Lucía noted that having a central hub for CHWs to congregate and share their experiences, concerns, challenges, and successes could serve as a system of support for the workforce. While she has noted that previous attempts to get CHWs to gather in the form of a "certification course class reunion" have been difficult, she explained, "It's very difficult to get them together but we know that they're out there changing the world." At the very least, creating the means for CHWs to gather, converse, and support one another is another system of support that can be offered to facilitate self-care and prevent and/or diminish burnout. Lucía expanded on her recommendations as well noting that she has seen that the caseload for CHWs is typically very high. She suggested creating policy or guidelines to serve as a system of support, or potentially tailoring caseload per individual CHW to best suit their capabilities. She also suggested having paid mental health days or even a mental health hour to allow the CHW to recharge and thus avoid the buildup of burnout.

Understanding the systems of support that are needed, especially as described by the CHWs themselves, is essential for policy-makers, employers, and other stakeholders to understand in order to help support these workers, prevent burnout and compassion fatigue, and provide support for self-care practices. During follow-up research completed in the summer of 2019, I spoke with Carmen again. I asked her what has been her solution to dealing with burnout, and she candidly replied, "I'm ending this job." She went on to discuss, as she did in the previous section, that the lack of infrastructure, internal support, heavy client load, and medical interpreting had become too much for her. Her example serves as a microcosm of what could easily happen if the concerns and calls for support from CHWs go unheeded underscoring how stakeholders must hear the needs of these workers.

"I CAN'T TAKE IT HOME": STRATEGIES OF SELF-CARE AMONG CHWS

Self-care is defined by the World Health Organization (WHO) as "the ability of individuals, families and communities to promote health, prevent disease, maintain health, and to cope with illness and disability with or without the support of a healthcare provider."[26] This practice can be achieved through a variety of means, including hygiene, nutrition, environmental factors (e.g., living conditions, habits, etc.), socioeconomic factors (e.g., income, cultural beliefs, etc.), and self-medication.[27] The WHO also describes self-care as being broader than just the individual, which is attained through self-reliance, empowerment, and autonomy but also within the greater community (i.e. achieved through community participation, community involvement, and community empowerment). In these ways, self-care serves to diminish stress enacted due to burnout and compassion fatigue but also establish healthy boundaries between work and personal life. This being especially important for CHWs who occupy this liminal professional citizenship within the broader moral economy of care.

The need to maintain mental and emotional well-being through self-care was vital in order to provide care to clients and effectively work as CHWs. Moreover, the looming issue of burnout and compassion fatigue made it all the more important for participants to not only preserve their well-being but also avoid these threats as well. At an institutional level, the certification course emphasized skills such as knowing when to remove yourself from a situation, discovering strategies to practice self-care, and ensuring self-care is practiced by CHWs. In our interview, Marcellus related to me that self-care is "very, very important. You cannot pour from an empty cup."

Participants varied widely when it came to the practice of self-care. There were some activities that were common in responses among participants, including relying on spirituality, prayer, meditation, reading, exercise, journaling, yoga, eating healthy, hiking, camping, having "me" time, taking time for self-reflection, seeing a therapist, and spending time with family members. Isabella explained her self-care routine, stating, "And I'm more aware of having my alone time.... I'll have quiet time where I just kinda sit out and listen to the birds and, you know, just take deep breaths and that's my little self-care. In evenings, going to walk. And just by myself or just have some quiet reading time that helps me just kind of release all the negative things around me." Other participants relied on their religiosity as a form of self-care. Lucía explained two strategies she uses to prevent buildup of compassion fatigue and burnout. She relies on her spirituality and her relationship with God. But "in the rigor of the day," as she described, Lucía takes time for herself, sometimes as little as 30 minutes, to go out into nature, get fresh air, and meditate. She emphasized taking time for herself in those stressful moments even for just 30 minutes can help her get through the day. Thus, for many CHWs, taking time to slow down and remove themselves from the daily stresses of work were key strategies of self-care.

Self-Care at Work

These participants had integrated self-care with their technology during the day. Rhonda, a CHW and case manager, developed a strategy in which she would put automated notifications in her work calendar that would remind her to take time during the day to practice self-care. Over the years, Andrés became skillful at scheduling his clients to not only maximize his efficiency and effectiveness as a CHW but also preserve his own mental health through making a schedule that worked best for him. In both of these examples, the CHWs integrated self-care into their daily work schedules as a strategy to help get through each day.

Other participants also integrated self-care routines into their daily work schedule. I drove to a large city in northern Indiana to interview a small team of CHWs in August 2017. I was shown around their office, learned about the various neighborhoods they served, and interviewed each CHW one-on-one. They also invited me to have lunch with them, which I later learned was something they also do regularly as a group. In fact, I was told, it was practically a requirement. During my interview with Marcia, I asked her about self-care and how it is practiced within their organization, she explained:

> Well, we laugh a lot and... don't take things so seriously. And we also do a lot of meditation and provide time for people to just rest. I encourage my people to actually have a meal together. I encourage them to not eat at their desks. I don't allow my staff to eat at their desks. You need to get up and walk away from the issue, spend some time walking around the building, so you have to care for yourself. So those are some of the things we do. We laugh. But you probably noticed that.

I remarked that I enjoyed eating at what felt like a "family meal." I also brought up the social cohesion shared between her and the CHWs. Marcia added:

Oh yeah, we do that all the time and the reason why we do that is because most of the people are single and they eat by themselves all the time but . . . I'm married and so is Margaret . . . and so Beverly is the only one that is not and she eats a lot by herself and she's like "No,"—when it comes to lunch time she's like— "I'm not eating by myself." So, it's a family thing and we have been doing that for many, many years. Everybody eats together, even when we bring our lunch, we all eat together. And you learn a lot about a person when you eat together at the table and we laugh a lot.

This informal and daily self-care support group provides a framework for these CHWs to acknowledge one another and provide a sense of comfort. Especially as Marcia notes, it's important for her employees to get away from their desks and fully disconnect from their work. Moreover, it diminishes stress that can be enacted through bottling up work-life tension through socialization with coworkers and feeling valued in the workplace.[28] Unfortunately, this seemed to be the exception rather than the rule among CHWs in the sample as many were the only CHW employed at the organization. However, this could serve as an example of the benefits of instituting a formal CHW support group, either by region in the state and/or a state-wide support group—especially to deter the buildup of burnout and compassion fatigue.

The Connection between Self-Care and Caregiving

Marcia explained the connection between the well-being of CHWs and how it directly relates to their caregiving, stating, "The ability for you to be healthy as well as the people you provide services too. And I say that because you are compassionate and you get so involved that you tend to forget that you need to be healthy and safe as well so I think that's one of the big issues that we are confronting all the time." Marcia echoed the earlier words of Alma and Beverly in describing their connection and commitment to their client can make them forget they too must care for their own health. Given their shared structural vulnerability, lack of professional citizenship, tenuous employment, and looming threats of burnout and compassion fatigue practicing self-care is a prominent and pertinent issue for CHWs to be effective in their caregiving.

Many participants in this study described having to "learn" to practice self-care. Participants told me that, in their first few years of work, they would make themselves available to clients at all times and, vicariously, adopt the health and social problems of their clients as their own. However, after several years, many CHWs described becoming savvier and more experienced and thus adjusted their approach to clients as one means of practicing self-care.

Juana, a CHW with more than a decade of experience, explained how adjusting your approach to care is one means of not only practicing self-care but also how the relationship between the CHW and client is intimately intertwined in this process. Juana told me that she had a client who she worked tirelessly to provide this individual with a variety of resources, options, and strategies to address their health issues yet engendering empowerment in this client remained elusive. As a result, she became frustrated and often reflected this failure on herself. However, she later realized that doing so was negatively affecting her ability to provide care to others and also draining her mental fortitude. Juana stated that distancing her life from her clients' issues was an essential means to practice self-care, preserve her own well-being, and maintain the stamina to help others:

> I have learned that their problems are not my problems [laughing] . . . I always say that . . . you cannot make their problems your own. You can give them the tools and I have done that . . . but at the end they need to use them. Like I said, I work with diabetes, we are in your boat and we are here helping you—or we can get out of the boat . . . it has to be a partnership. I will help you as long as you are willing to help yourself. . . . But I know that I cannot solve all of their problems so that is part of my own mental health.

Enacting a boundary by separating oneself from issues present with challenging clients was a strategy seen among other CHWs as well. Gabriela described practicing distancing oneself from clients who are continuing, deliberately, to engage in poor health choices. She asserted that a CHW must preserve their own mental and emotional well-being lest they risk diminishing their caregiving and own mental well-being. Distancing oneself from such a client, in this instance, becomes a strategy of self-care. Gabriela described this case:

> I have to be very able to go back and forth and in all of it understand that it's people's decisions. While my heart goes out to the individual who is dying that has made poor decisions and my heart goes out to an organization that is struggling, it's not my problem. I can't take it home, I can't own it, I do my best and I'm not going to lose any sleep over it . . . but it took me years to get to the point that I don't lose any sleep over it. After the first four or five years of doing this fulltime with my organization, I learned that it's not my [problem].

Gabriela elaborated how distancing oneself from specific problems of clients or organizations is necessary to not only maintain one's own mental well-being but also put that energy into helping other clients. She explained, "I can't be effective in a meeting if I'm boo-hooing about someone that I love dearly that is choosing to die. I can't function and advocate for the thirty-some patients that I need to advocate [for] if one has got me down like that. So it's learning to balance that." As such, moving on from particular clients and/or organizations not only respected autonomy but also served as a strategy for self-care that assuaged the CHWs' well-being in addition to preserving their capacity to be effective with other clients and situations.

Challenges in Practicing Self-Care

Despite the benefits and overall need for self-care, practicing it was a challenge for some CHWs. While CHWs engaged in advocacy for clients, they were unsure of how to participate in professional-level advocacy in terms of seeking help for their own needs. Not practicing self-care was also exacerbated by some participants who felt as though they were unable to slow down and take time for themselves, which resulted in a precarious cycle that bordered into burnout. Rosa, a CHW and a doula, related these challenges to me, "Sometimes we [CHWs] don't know how to talk to get these resources [for our self-care]." Mark highlighted the issues he has experienced trying to slow down, "Actually, I've often said I like doing nothing. But I don't do that very well at all. It's good in a way because we have lots of energy and if we can channel it, you can make a difference in the world but if it's a marathon instead of a sprint we're not going to be around for the long haul if we don't watch it." Thus, self-care could be hard for some participants and they could become trapped in a cycle in which a CHW was unsure how to ask for help and how to slow down.

The need to develop strategies of self-care was evident among this workforce not only to guard their own emotional and mental well-being but also to be able to effectively serve their clients and communities. In many ways, practicing self-care not only ensured the well-being of the CHW but also as a way to ensure efficacious care for clients. Within the moral economy of care, CHWs—serving as a conduit between structurally vulnerable populations and biomedicine—often placed the needs of their clients and community above that of their own and, thereby, sacrificed their own well-being.

Moreover, due to the taxing nature of this work on CHWs, they should be provided additional forms of care (e.g., access to mental health counselors, therapists) aside from simply practicing self-care. As Backe notes for rape crisis hotline operators, self-care could be "insufficient" and that "[self-care] accommodates the absence of formalized care structures for caregivers."[29] Providing CHWs with access to these other means to promote their well-being is essential to ensuring their own health and ability to provide care. Gabriela asserted that CHWs have a right to advocate for their needs just as they do for their clients, " . . . I think that that's a self-care element that maybe is ignored in this field that you do have a right to advocate for yourself and who your position is, as a CHW."

STAYING IN OR GETTING OFF THE BOAT: TOUGH LOVE AS PROMOTING SELF-CARE?

Tough love, or trying to get someone (often a loved one) to take responsibility for themselves to improve their situation in the long run via the enactment of constraints, was a divisive topic among CHWs. For some participants, this emerged as a strategy of self-care when dealing with a difficult client. Several participants explained that they have had to cut off a client in order to preserve their own mental and emotional well-being. When I asked Juana whether or not there was such a thing as tough love in CHW care, she explained, "Oh yes, yes, yes. And that's one of the things that is very important is to let them know '*You're* leading this boat. We're here to support you, but at the same time, we can get off.'" But, she also emphasized, "That can be done in a loving way." Others argued that cutting off a client was an impossibility—it rested with the CHW to continue to find ways to support the client or find another CHW who could help. However, in several of my conversations with CHWs, participants felt that tough love was an overreach of the CHWs' responsibilities. Tough love was something only to be exercised by family members or romantic partners. Others saw tough love as needing to distance themselves from a client and/or to simply remind clients that they themselves are in charge of their life. As such, sometimes participants had enacted boundaries between themselves and particularly challenging clients.

Martha explained that she believes that it is on the CHW to make the decision of ending care. She expounded that it is situationally driven but that a CHW can still provide care through referrals but can also decide to move on in order to help other clients. Martha stated, "And the CHW would need to know her client and know when to cut ties and just let go . . . as a CHW you cannot carry that person forever." Martha asserted, "And just giving them whatever resource referrals to help them if there are others out there that might be able [to help them] . . . because there's only so much the CHW can do." Recognizing that CHWs have limitations as well as professional boundaries with clients to maintain is vital to ensuring these workers do not have stress that can contribute to experiencing burnout and/or compassion fatigue.

Carmen also agreed that tough love absolutely exists in community health work. She explained that "sometimes you have to step back and realize the patient has to make these decisions. Man or woman up and deal with it . . . you're not doing them a service. It's almost [like] we've become enablers, I guess." Thus, according to Carmen, in failing to engender empowerment more damage can be done in not taking the necessary steps to practice tough love. As such, aside from experiencing stress from a client, which can contribute to burnout, participants could become intertwined in a relationship that enables the client's deleterious habits.

However, some participants were less keen on the concept of tough love at least professionally. In my conversations with Beverly, we spoke about whether or not tough love is a suitable approach to employ as a CHW. She recalled the scope of care as a fixture in stating, "Tough love is like—you're in a particular place where you're gonna have them tough it out. You're gonna stick to your guns. Well, you know, we have to stick to our scope of practice. Whatever your scope of practice is, that's what you stick to. So, I don't know if there's a whole lot of tough love in that." Beverly elaborated that tough love should not be in the CHW repertoire, "Because I don't think . . . a community health worker can do tough love. Because I think when you do tough love, you're taking it out of the clients' hands . . . so you have to be very careful about that. When we're talking about client-centered, that's not part of it."

As such, practicing tough love, to some participants, was essentially antithetical to being a CHW. While CHWs must adhere to their scope of care, that in and of itself prohibits tough love. CHW work is defined by this scope and, in operating in said scope, CHWs do not practice tough love. However, at least for the CHWs who agreed that tough love is necessary, doing so addresses issues in scope of care that would not provide guidelines for these situations. Thus, cutting off a client might be one way to aid their own mental well-being. Alma was also against the use of tough love when it came to clients, explaining:

No, no . . . In my own personal opinion, tough love is reserved for someone that you really, really know very, very well and know that they'll blossom with that and that they're gonna take that and... they're gonna show you that they can do it. At least, again, that's my experience. With clients that you're working with, with people that you're trying to establish a relationship with so that they can trust you, so that they know that you're the first one to go to. I really don't see the tough love aspect working very well because, again, you don't know each other very well. . . . It's usually those first couple of meetings that you have with clients that are really, again, gonna have them say, "Yes, I wanna go back." Or, "No, this person was just a total jerk and I really don't feel like dealing with this on top of everything else that I have to deal with." So, yeah, I, the tough love thing, I really don't believe in that. I don't.

Other CHWs were also skeptical about cutting someone off or practicing tough love. "But tough love can be misguided too," Marcellus cautioned.

When encountering a client who does not seem to want to become empowered, Marcellus tends to practice other strategies to reach the client. While he noted he may need to "back up" and remove himself from the situation, he would come back to help out at a later time. He explained, "I let people look into my life." In particular, he would share with them his ten-year experience with homelessness, his previous hospitalizations, and his twelve years of sobriety. Thus, instead of practicing tough love, he takes a different approach by inviting clients into his life experience and see how he has overcome difficult situations.

Rather than tough love, other CHWs stressed accountability. Leticia asserted that CHWs should hold clients accountable and emphasized that caregiving provided by these workers must be client-driven and client-centered. Tough love is not inherent within this form of care, rather these workers should ask clients "Why?" and "What's going on?" in order to determine the issues for why they are not being accountable and provide space for clients to practice autonomy over their health issues. In this way, CHWs could try new angles to determine why a client is not becoming empowered and might also discover new strategies to provide care and thereby reduce the stress experienced with clients who do not seem to want to become empowered.

Finally, Gabriela noted that CHWs should be practicing healthy boundaries with clients. Individuals who might push a CHW and not practice autonomy can have negative mental health repercussions by creating a stressful situation for the CHW. She viewed tough love as a power imbalance, in which the CHW has power over the client. Rather, she argued, CHWs should always be transferring that power to the client. Instead, Gabriela asserted, "You want to respect people and where they're at. So, you have to acknowledge that it protects the CHW not to push." Maintaining healthy boundaries protects CHWs from these potentially stressful positions with clients without also straying into issues of power imbalance by practicing tough love. She contrasted this with a comparison to the experience of a parent with a child, one in which the parent is always going to be there for their child, while a CHW must maintain professional boundaries. Instead, she stated, "Whereas, what I'm suggesting is that we just have *influence* and be and let be."

SUPPORTING SELF-CARE

Although some CHWs were adept at managing their well-being through various self-care routines, it took some participants years to develop this practice and others only did so after coming close to or directly experiencing burnout. Furthermore, many of these strategies were highly and, unsurprisingly, individualized and mostly conducted outside of work. While some strategies discussed were implemented within the workplace, such as lunches together, other options should be considered and implemented to protect and care for the mental and emotional needs of CHWs. Lucía, Isabella, and other participants have noted the need for professional forms of self-care, such as a central hub for CHWs in the state to connect, network, and converse with other CHWs in addition to implementing and providing adequate breaks (such as a "mental health hour") or specific paid time off to support their mental health needs.

The need for wider action on support for self-care of CHWs was also a topic during the focus group interview. When presenting the initial findings from the research, there was a discussion among the participants related to self-care. The general consensus was that more needs to be done to help CHWs institute self-care and provide alternative forms of support. Networking in this way, as participants suggested, would provide means to meet and speak with other CHWs while also serving as a place where others can seek support. These workers also suggested implementing routines such as having a state-wide, CHW self-care meeting at least every 3 months.

CHWOI is also organizationally supporting CHWs in developing strategies for practicing self-care. Lucía explained that CHWOI is drawing on the mind-body medicine already in use in California and on the East Coast. This strategy draws on a mixture of principles and practices including intentionality, yoga, and relaxation to address stressful situations. Lucía explained that not only will this self-care practice help CHWs, but that these workers can also pass on this strategy to their clients as a strategy to overcome stressful situations. Previous research has demonstrated positive effects in teaching CHWs stress coping mechanisms who responded to the aftermath of Hurricane Sandy.[30] Training these workers in this method helped to reduce rates of burnout and improve the overall work environment.[31]

Major organizations such as the WHO[32] have described several important benefits that can be ascertained through supporting self-care initiatives including strengthening institutions to maximize efficient use of domestic health resources, creating health sector innovations, and improving overall access to medicines and interventions through the optimal interfacing of health systems and sites of healthcare delivery. Instituting these initiatives can help CHWs and their counterparts stay mentally and emotionally healthy, deliver efficacious care to clients.

Overall, instituting self-care practices must be maintained and supported by policy-makers, employers, and organizations and be practiced by the workers themselves. CHWs must be provided with support and the means to practice self-care (in addition to being encouraged to do so). Organizations and employers should consider setting up a support group whether in person, virtual, or both options so that CHWs can come together and support one another. Implementing various strategies as an organization or employer, such as the mind-body medicine employed by CHWOI, should be implemented to provide a variety of strategies to practice self-care. In doing so, CHWs can maintain their physical and mental well-being while also being able to effectively care for those in their service.

STEPS FORWARD: DIMINISHING BURNOUT AND COMPASSION FATIGUE AND INSTITUTIONALIZING SELF-CARE

The broader political economic environment and moral economy of care impact the well-being of CHWs. Due to their structural and professional vulnerabilities, coupled with the great needs of their clients and communities, many participants described placing their own well-being second to that of those in need. While some CHWs have developed strategies of self-care to avoid sacrificing their state of mind and physical health, others are still suffering from these various issues. Failure to address self-care can lead to burnout and compassion fatigue.

Burnout and compassion fatigue are deleterious conditions that compromise the ability of CHWs (and other healthcare workers) to provide care efficaciously. Especially for CHWs who must maintain their position within the moral economy of care, burnout and compassion fatigue compromise their ability to not only provide care but also function in this position. As CHWs have previously noted, breakdowns in the relationship between CHW and client can cause irreparable damage. Alma provided an additional example of how burnout compromises her ability to provide care for her clients but also how CHWs can turn these negative experiences, whether it's their own or those of other clients, into a positive:

> It's like . . . if you burn out completely, you're not gonna be able to do much for anyone. So, you have to keep going and you have to use these experiences as almost testimonies . . . to encourage others that may be seeking something like this either as a client or as a CHW. Just because we've gone through our fair share of negative experiences, doesn't mean that we can't turn them into [something] positive.

Policy-makers, (potential) employers, and other stakeholders must realize the impacts of burnout and compassion fatigue and work to support CHWs as they are integrated into the workforce. Especially given the fact that CHWs face structural and professional vulnerability, offering aid and self-care options is vital in order for these workers to effectively serve their populations.

Tough love, a strategy of self-care for some participants, was a divisive topic. While some asserted that it was a viable strategy to use with participants, others argued that it crossed a professional boundary and is something that is only practiced with family members and loved ones. For the participants that utilized the strategy of tough love, it served to protect their mental well-being and promote self-care when a client was not taking the necessary steps to own their health behaviors. Others stressed accountability on part of the client and finding other angles from which to serve the client and, if necessary, stepping back and referring the client elsewhere to protect their mental well-being.

Although employers and other stakeholders have little influence over the self-care routines outside of work, they must take time to institute self-care practices in the workplace.[33] Taking steps to develop a CHW support group or network are other options to provide additional channels for networking and self-care with other CHWs. In 2020, CHWOI began holding live, self-care online events for CHWs throughout the state each month. Providing these resources, both for self-care at work and self-care outside of work are essential in order to provide "care for the carers" especially as these workers undergo professionalization. In doing so, these workers will maximize their well-being and service to their clients. Policy-makers, employers, and other stakeholders can support the ability of CHWs to practice self-care and thus promote their own mental well-being.

Supporting CHWs through a variety of means outlined throughout the chapter is vital for helping to not only integrate these workers but also to ensure that they themselves are cared for within the workforce. Employers must recognize the role of CHWs within the moral economy of care, the impact of workplace stresses, the nuances of their relationships with clients, and support the needs of these workers to ensure their well-being as they provide care. In doing so, policy-makers, employers, and other stakeholders can care for the workforce and prevent burnout and compassion fatigue from compromising the caregiving of CHWs.

NOTES

1. Adams et al. 2006, De Hert 2020.
2. Motta 2008: 291.
3. These are not classified as medical conditions (WHO 2019).
4. Burnout occurs due to workplace stressors overtime whereas compassion fatigue is caused by exposure to traumatic material. For more information on the differences between these two factors, see https://www.griefworkcenter.com/compassion-fatigue-vs-burnout/.
5. It is important to note that burnout can occur in any profession (De Hert 2020).
6. De Hert 2020: 171.

7. Ibid.
8. De Hert 2020, Bhutani et al. 2012, WHO 2019.
9. De Hert 2020, WHO 2019.
10. De Hert 2020.
11. Turgoose and Maddox 2017: 172.
12. Ligenza 2018.
13. Ibid.
14. Backe 2018, Besterman-Dahan et al. 2014.
15. Berthold 2016.
16. Ibid.
17. Alkema et al. 2008, Coaston 2017, Horn and Johnston 2020, Lawson and Cook 2017, Salloum et al. 2015, Sansó et al. 2015.
18. Maslach and Leiter 2017, Kleinpell et al. 2020.
19. See, e.g., Bijari and Abassi 2016, Haq et al. 2008, Malakouti et al. 2011, Mota et al. 2014, Selamu et al. 2017, Tantchou 2014, Tripathy et al. 2016.
20. Ge et al. 2011, Li et al. 2014.
21. Lo and Nguyen 2021, Russ 2005.
22. Lo and Nguyen 2021: 7.
23. Mota et al. 2014.
24. De Hert 2020.
25. Tripathy et al. 2016.
26. WHO 2020.
27. Ibid.
28. Horn and Johnston 2020.
29. Backe 2018: 475.
30. Powell and Yuma-Guerrero 2016.
31. Mota et al. 2014, Powell and Yuma-Guerrero 2016.
32. WHO 2020.
33. Powell and Yuma-Guerrero 2016.

Conclusion

Well, we believe that CHWs are the new way of assisting and providing
healthcare services to all populations, but especially populations of
color, because we see the increased number of people in America—
and America is changing. People want to be cared for and educated
by people that look like them, and this is a good way to increase
employment for the population that we are serving, it is a good way
to integrate the healthcare system to make it more like the population
that we serve, and it is an excellent way to provide services to all
populations.

—Marcia, CHW

Marcia related this to me during my trip to visit their CHW organization in
northeastern Indiana. She adeptly explained many of the benefits—current
and potential—of CHWs. As Marcia notes, CHWs extend care to not only
all populations but especially for populations of color who experience racism, marginalization, and structural violence. Marcia also notes the impact of
shared race and ethnicity in stating, "people want to be cared for and educated
by people that look like them," a key facet that established and deepened the
CHW-client relationship within the moral economy of care. Job development
via the professional incorporation of these workers also represents an opportunity within these communities. While CHWs traverse boundaries in care,
they also face many barriers. However, the healthcare needs of communities
in Indiana—and throughout the United States—underscore the need for these
workers.

This book has explored the lived experiences of CHWs through the lens
of medical anthropology. While many studies exist regarding these workers
in the United States, few have deeply examined the quotidian experiences,

the nuances in their relationships with stakeholders and clients, and assessed issues of professionalization in the nascency of their integration. A key contribution of this book is elevating the voices of the participants and involving them within the project to bring their experiences to the forefront. This book has sought to amplify the voices of these workers, their professional needs, their experiences in providing care, and the contexts of the environment in which they work and the state of their communities. As such, these stories and lived experiences can inform and enlighten policy development related to this workforce. In this way, the participants and myself have sought to demystify their *present yet invisible* nature in the workforce and underscore their unique contributions and requisite nature of their caregiving.

Although CHWs have existed within the United States since the 1960s, they have often functioned on the periphery of the healthcare and social services workforces. However, CHWs have provided much-needed care, resources, and advocacy for marginalized populations throughout the country. This book detailed the lived experiences of these workers in Indiana, the issues they encountered, and how their professionalization has played out since 2017. This book also demonstrates that the landscape in which CHWs operate is one intimately entangled within larger, political economic forces that shape and mold the livelihood and caregiving provided by these workers within the moral economy of care. Previous anthropological studies have assessed these issues and caregiving among other paraprofessionals and how structural forces affect caregivers and clients.[1] The findings presented in the book contribute to these studies in elucidating the lived experiences, unique roles, and challenges encountered by CHWs.

Although there are an estimated 56,130[2] CHWs employed throughout the United States (and an estimated 1,270 in Indiana[3]), many remain on the fringes of the healthcare system. The shortage of healthcare workers in the United States[4] and abroad[5] and, especially, in rural areas[6] highlights opportunities for CHWs and their counterparts.[7] The U.S. Bureau of Labor Statistics predicts this field will experience an 11 percent increase from 2018 to 2028, which notes that this growth is due to "efforts to improve health outcomes" and "to reduce healthcare costs."[8] This is to be specifically achieved through health education in helping clients understand how to utilize healthcare services.[9] Moreover, the COVID-19 pandemic has laid bare weaknesses in healthcare systems[10] and exacerbated health inequities including unequal morbidity and mortality rates among populations of color,[11] which become exacerbated via discrimination, racism, and the social determinants of health.[12] Public health professionals, scholars, and health organizations are again calling for their incorporation into the workforce as one means to address these deleterious and structural factors in addition to new ways forward in imagining the health workforce—with CHWs as key players.[13]

Through health education, advocacy, informal counseling, engendering empowerment, and increasing access to care and resources, these workers circumvent the deleterious effects of social determinants of health. This results in improved health outcomes for clients and communities and reduced costs for the healthcare system by aiding populations manage chronic conditions, successfully adhere to treatment plans, and reduce rates of hospital readmission. Martha echoed these sentiments in identifying CHWs as "gatekeepers," stating, "CHWs are supporting and being a gatekeeper at the front end so that these individual clients don't go back into the system." CHWs, as such, open the gates to care and aid clients in managing their health conditions and overcoming deleterious structural forces.

In this final portion of the book, I not only present summations and syntheses of the major themes but also include several dilemmas and potential for barriers and boundaries that may emerge for these workers. Additionally, I outline the applied contributions from the research presented in this book. I also describe areas for future research that will not only illuminate academic insights but will also, ideally, yield applicable findings. Conducting research with CHWs in the United States—and abroad—is an area rich for collaboration and highlighting the lived experiences and contributions of these workers.[14] Continuing to work in this capacity with CHWs in the United States and abroad will not only yield theoretical and academic contributions but, most importantly, findings that inform policy, create salubrious public (and global) health impacts, and positively shape the professional experience of these workers.

SYNTHESIZING CARE, RELATIONSHIPS, AND POLICY WITHIN THE MORAL ECONOMY OF CARE

The stories and experiences presented in this book reveal the intricate entanglement of a variety of actors (e.g., CHWs, clients, executive directors, politicians), policies, and organizations that influence and mold the moral economy of care. The lens of moral economy elucidates how law, policy, rhetoric, morals, values, and actors (e.g., policy-makers) shape access to care and provision of resources and, thereby, structure the relationships between actors at the ground level. Other studies have utilized this theoretical framework to produce applied findings for policy and practice for healthcare workers (including CHWs), those receiving care, and within healthcare systems.[15]

Moral economy sheds light into the relationships between CHWs and clients. Building trust and nurturing a relationship centered around understanding and compassion were essential. Shared race, ethnicity, culture, gender, and/or language were leveraged by participants to establish connections in addition to speaking from shared experience, thereby removing barriers and crossing boundaries in fostering relationships with clients. This relationship was centered on moral obligation and motivation on the part of the CHW to serve and provide care to their clients and communities.

Understanding the motivations, values, and morals of CHWs and how their care is affected by the political economic context can and must inform policy and legislation on CHWs and relevant public health programs. In the same vein of Bourgois,[16] Bourgois and Schonberg,[17] and Horton,[18] understanding the relations, norms, and social obligations that include or exclude the actors within these various moral economies is vital to implementing effective public policy and public health programs. Zabiliūtė asserts,

> For anthropologists, the task is to go beyond the assumption that the relationships of CHWs with their communities are given, and to explore the kinds of relationships that exist in specific contexts, over the course of time, and the ways that relationalities that cannot be contained or predefined by such programs are maintained and lived by.[19]

The findings produced by drawing on the lens of moral economy can directly inform policy development by elucidating how care, relationships, and policy mold the political economic context and how relationships are fostered, structured, and nurtured between CHWs and clients.[20]

DIFFICULTIES IN ENGENDERING EMPOWERMENT AND SELF-SUFFICIENCY IN THE MORAL ECONOMY OF CARE

Empowering clients to take ownership of their health was a core component of the CHW-client relationship. Via engendering empowerment, CHWs sought to unlock self-sufficiency within the client to overcome barriers and boundaries to enhance their overall well-being. However, several participants noted challenges from clients who seemingly did not want to become empowered and achieve self-sufficiency. While guiding, teaching, and coaching were anticipated as the initial steps for CHWs in helping clients, there was an expectation that clients would slowly take more and more of an active lead in the various issues they navigated with CHWs. Thus, this central aspect of the CHW-client relationship couched within the moral economy was one in which the worker invested their moral obligation, time, energy, and resources as a means to engender empowerment within their client. Participants noted that even if their client developed self-sufficiency, they would always be there to help them should the need arise.

However, engendering empowerment is also entangled with the neoliberal approach to care, which centers on health and health behaviors being solely the responsibility of the individual. This becomes especially difficult for the populations served by CHWs given their structurally vulnerable positions in society, experiences with discrimination and racism, and unequal access to care and opportunities. As discussed in chapter 1, although CHWs extend the medical gaze from the clinic into their communities, they also soften its impact through their advocacy, compassion, and continual support of their communities and clients. Much like Nading's[21] analysis of the dualistic role of CHWs within the moral economy, participants were at once extending the reach of biomedicine but also serving as compassionate neighbors and agents of change. Likewise, CHWs soften the reach of the neoliberal approach in their caregiving by serving as accessible aides while also advocating for change at the macro level.

CHWs experienced difficulties with particular clients, especially those who failed to reach (or show steady improvement toward) empowerment breached this core component of the CHW-client relationship. CHWs, who invested their time, knowledge, and resources, expected that their clients would become empowered. Participants struggled to determine when enough was enough or whether or not they should cut someone off. Participants, such as Isabella, struggled with this, often taking it as a personal failing related to her work as a CHW rather than blaming the client. There was not a clear answer in how to proceed, with CHWs taking it as a failure on their part, others continuing to help clients, and yet others sought to find another CHW who might better help the said client.

Maintaining positive relationships and their reputation within the moral economy was essential for CHWs. Beverly noted the negative repercussions of a poor referral or failure to secure resources in terms of damaging the CHW's reputation within the community. Cutting off an individual could provoke negative repercussions and cause these workers to lose rapport and respect. Given their deep connection within the community and possible overlap in network between clients, taking such action could be precarious. However, participants were faced with their own health issues in choosing to continue to provide care for such clients—experiencing frustration and feelings of failure deleteriously impacts the CHW's mental health and well-being. For many participants, there was no easy answer and was on a case-by-case basis.

Employer guidelines and scope of care may help with determining when to move on from a troubling client. Gabriela summed up the potential negative impacts in chapter 6, explaining that if she's too caught up in issues related to someone who is choosing to make poor health decisions, she will be unable to be effective in helping others who are truly set on becoming a healthy and self-sufficient client. Thus, at least one solution is present, if the individual is actively choosing poor health decisions (and/or refusing to take steps toward self-sufficiency) then the CHW must move on to other clients.

CONSIDERATIONS FOR POLICY
DEVELOPMENT AND CHW LEADERSHIP

The CHW task force was convened by the governor of Indiana to professionalize CHWs and develop policy related to the model and for Medicaid reimbursement with the explicit goal for these workers to improve health outcomes throughout Indiana. However, CHW representation in this task force was lacking, with Lucía being the only CHW among a varied group of stakeholders (who were mostly White). This fact underscores how women, and women of color in particular, have been excluded from and within the professional realm[22] and is indicative of the precarious position of CHWs in general in Indiana. Despite the convening of the task force aimed to ameliorate health issues through the professionalization of CHWs, the initial conception of these workers and issues related to their core responsibilities and contributions to the workforce were far from the reality. However, it must be noted that members of the task force were genuinely interested in the model and were eager to properly develop the position.

As Lucía was the only CHW on the committee, she bore the brunt of the work—truly functioning in her CHW capacity, and participating in professional-level advocacy—by educating the other members of what a CHW is and their core roles and contributions. Her participation in this task force, much as Beverly's and Andrés's participation in community coalitions, underscores the unpaid labor that CHWs undertake to promote their position and needs of their fellow CHWs and communities.

Critical advancements of the task force included the policy development related to the core competencies of CHWs in Indiana as well as Medicaid reimbursement. As noted earlier, offering reimbursement for activities that are strictly biomedical focused may overmedicalize the position and devalue roles (such as advocacy) that are social-focused but directly related to engendering empowerment and ameliorating health issues encountered by clients outside of the clinic. While participants told me that the reimbursement rates have been low through 2021, the overarching impacts of having solely biomedical services reimbursable remains to be seen. And especially in terms of how they may impact and shift the type of care and activities CHWs participate in.

While laws, such as the ACA, made important strides in terms of recognizing the CHW workforce, there have been little advancements in sustainable funding (and institutionalized salaries) in addition to further guidance for the integration of the workforce. Several successful examples of such programs exist in Arizona, Massachusetts, Minnesota, and Oregon, of which have highlighted the unique roles of CHWs including cultural humility, improvements to quality of care, and cost-effectiveness.[23]

In particular, Massachusetts created the Office of Community Health Workers that oversees workforce surveillance, standardization and implementation of training, and policy development within the state.[24] Minnesota is one state that has made a "full spectrum" of CHW services reimbursable through Medicaid.[25] These two states serve as a model for other states to analyze when implementing a successful CHW program—both in terms of legislation and policy development, as well as reimbursement. Steps that integrate these workers must assess the utility of their roles as both basic healthcare providers, as advocates, and including them in policy development related to their position.[26] These examples highlight how a partnership can successfully function between state public health officials and community health workers in facilitating a successful integration of this workforce.

Rosenthal et al.[27] assert that four primary policy recommendations serve as the impetus for the creation of a CHW workforce. These include (1) creation of sustainable funding for CHW services through Medicaid, Children's Health Insurance Program (CHIP), and other funding sources; (2) offering workforce development through a variety of trainings and options for career development; (3) regulation of the position through standardized training and certification; and (4) development of a common set of measures to assess CHWs and their provided services. Rosenthal et al. also assert that CHWs be involved in shaping policy that affects their position as well as providing options to minimize the cost of trainings and reducing other barriers to employment including language, citizenship, life experiences, and education.

In addition to these policy and public health program implications, other stakeholders (e.g., politicians, nongovernmental organizations, employers, and potential employers) have an obligation to reach out to CHWs and establish leadership positions in discussions of their future. In doing so, differences between how stakeholders' visions regarding the CHW workforce and the actual experiences of these workers can be addressed between these actors unlike issues seen in other anthropological research on this topic.[28] As I asserted in chapter 3, politicians, public health officials, and other stakeholders should reach out to CHWs and involve them in steps that will legislate and define their professionalization and ability to provide caregiving. The inclusion of CHWs in policy-making is not new, with the American Public Health Association's (APHA) CHW Section[29] and the C3 Project[30] asserting the need for CHW leadership with support also found within the scholarly literature.[31] CHWs must be given ownership in decisions involving the direction of their profession.

ENHANCING PROFESSIONAL CITIZENSHIP: CERTIFICATION, MEDICAID REIMBURSEMENT, TERMINOLOGY, AND RAMIFICATIONS

As described in chapter 3, lacking professional citizenship is a major barrier that inhibits the integration of CHWs within the broader professional workforce. However, the introduction of two primary legitimizing mechanisms, certification and Medicaid reimbursement, were essential steps toward fostering the professional citizenship of these workers. Although these were important steps, they come with careful considerations and largely function as double-edged swords due to the changes and barriers they can provoke. Still, participants noted that professionalization is crucial for the advancement of CHWs in Indiana and in many other areas throughout the world.

While the certification may function as a legitimizing mechanism, it may manifest new barriers to entering the workforce for some (e.g., not being able to take time off and/or not having the finances to pay for the tuition), fostering a CHW hierarchy (between those with and without the certification), and for those who are unable to become employed with the certification (e.g., undocumented immigrants). Some participants were also ambivalent regarding the certification. CHWs who already had extensive experience felt as though their skills were reinforced, the certification did little to offer something new. However, other participants were in agreement that the certification would produce more legitimacy and acceptance regarding the CHW position. These participants described how the training advanced their personal growth which, in turn, allowed them to function more effectively as a CHW.

Medicaid reimbursement also functions as a legitimizing mechanism and is directly linked to the certification. Employers can claim reimbursement for the CHW-specific services so as long as their CHW is certified. Together, the certification and reimbursement address the issue of terminology regarding this position (see figure 3.1, chapter 3) since the specific verbiage in the policy states that only "community health workers" who have been certified are eligible for reimbursement. The majority of participants told me that they felt as though the general public, medical professionals, and social service organizations were unaware of the CHW position. The extensive titles used for these workers in Indiana have complicated its recognition within the public and professional spheres. Participants who worked behind the scenes during the rollout of the certification course and professionalization of the position were well aware of the issue related to terminology. The certification course, Medicaid reimbursement, and plans to have a CHW marketing campaign are potential solutions to addressing the lack of awareness. Increasing awareness may serve as another legitimizing mechanism that will enhance the legitimacy and professional citizenship of these workers. However, the issue of namebranding lingers in the state and it remains to be seen if these steps will result in current employers re-titling their workers as "[certified] community health workers."

In regards to the certification course, the classes were still in their nascency at the time of data collection. Many classes have occurred in the years since its initial rollout. There had been discussions related to refining specific classes within the training and augmenting with other topics. As noted earlier, some participants, particularly those who had prior experience as CHWs, wanted more specific technical and/or specialty trainings within the class. While the course was designed as a foundational level training, additional courses can be taken for these specialty courses. The primary concept was to retrain experienced CHWs and have all new CHWs go through the same training so that a baseline model could be constructed in the state and demonstrate that CHWs have earned the same certification.

Others steps can be taken to enhance the legitimacy of CHWs within the healthcare workforce, particularly as a means to increase positive health outcomes. Expanding the roles of CHWs employed as medical interpreters to allow additional positive health outcomes, especially via advocacy and ensuring the patient fully understands the diagnosis, prognosis, and treatment plan. Carmen provided the example of stepping outside her scope of care as a medical interpreter in questioning the doctor regarding the prescribed medication. This served, as Carmen explained, as a double-check for the doctor to ensure their prescription would be the lowest-cost alternative for the patient (and thus carry out the treatment plan as prescribed).

While the state government of Indiana came on board with the concept of these workers as a means to increase the health and well-being of the population, it must work with stakeholders to increase awareness, build acceptance, and establish systems of support for CHWs as they enter the workforce. The majority of CHWs come from and work within marginalized communities that are most in need of health and social services as well as advocacy. Their clients and broader communities lack medical citizenship due to structural violence and racism and have been deemed undeserving of care (e.g., especially those who are undocumented or are experiencing homelessness and/or substance use disorders). By enhancing the roles of CHWs within the broader workforce, these workers can produce significant impacts to improve the health equity of their communities. Ensuring that CHWs have professional citizenship will facilitate their success—with careful consideration for ramifications arising from professionalization.

ESTABLISHING HEALTHY BOUNDARIES: LAWS, POLICIES, SCOPE OF CARE, AND FUNDING

Although boundaries of care were established via a scope of care, this often resulted in a gray area for CHWs. As previously noted, the ambiguity of the CHW model is at once a strength and a weakness. The flexibility allows employers and CHWs to be adaptable to the ever-changing issues encountered by these workers within the community and shift to fill gaps in care. However, it was also difficult for some participants due to not having firm guidelines to follow. Nonetheless, scope of care, in addition to laws such as the HIPAA and employer and organizational guidelines, established boundaries and other times explicit barriers for CHWs to follow while providing care.

For some participants, these boundaries were crossed in the pursuit of care. Crossing these boundaries was morally justified, since participants were placing the health needs of the client at the forefront. Meanwhile, other participants would never think of crossing such boundaries and rather remained within these boundaries as a means to protect their health and profession. Going outside of scope was a divisive topic among participants that also echoed closely to issues encountered when a client wanted to participate in an activity that crossed a moral boundary with CHWs.

The line was increasingly blurred by CHWs who worked as medical interpreters. Due to the CHW position not being widely recognized in the professional workforce, many participants instead found employment as medical interpreters. However, serving as an interpreter was frustrating since they were technically not to interject or advocate on behalf of the client in the medical encounter. Some participants did cross this boundary, advocating to the client or clandestinely aiding them before or after the appointment. Carmen, for example, explained that the medical professional could actually be quite approving since it would remind the professional to look for cheaper medications or become aware of the structural issues that could impede the patient from adhering to the treatment plan.

In order to reinforce these boundaries and also look for opportunities, potential employers and employers should recognize the benefits of hiring a CHW and especially a CHW who can function as an interpreter and advocate for the patient, potentially ensuring enhanced quality of care. However, it is essential that they are remunerated appropriately, especially if taking on both of these roles within one job. Proper funding of CHW positions, increased salaries, and expanding the reach of these workers will help CHWs provide optimum care while also being compensated justly. Boundaries and barriers to entering the profession, remaining within the profession, and providing care must be examined and addressed to ensure the success of this workforce.

RECOGNIZING AND PRESERVING ADVOCACY AS CAREGIVING

Closely tied within the steps to professionalize and provide professional citizenship is preserving the core CHW role of advocacy, which serves as a unique function performed by these workers and has many direct impacts on health and well-being. Steps must be taken to ensure that advocacy remains a core function of the CHW model and particularly in policy development. As argued in chapter 5, advocacy must be understood, and reconceptualized, as a form of caregiving. I argue that CHWs engage in three distinct levels of advocacy at the micro, macro, and professional. In assessing the impact of advocacy in this way, policy-makers and (potential) employers can understand the various levels of impact that CHWs affect health and well-being. However, enhancing the role of CHWs in the professional workforce in Indiana has jeopardized their ability to participate in advocacy. As noted by other scholars, the professionalization of the CHW model often risks overmedicalizing their approach at the cost of their ability to perform advocacy.[32]

Advocacy within the CHW model has been a central pillar since its rise in Latin America in the 1950s and 1960s in conjunction with Catholic liberation theology[33] and the philosophies of Paulo Freire (e.g., *educação popular* [popular education]).[34] Advocacy not only addresses socioeconomic injustices but is also directly tied to the facilitation of care. Steps taken (especially in policy development) to limit, diminish, or end their ability to participate in advocacy would reposition the model toward biomedicine entirely—one cautioned by Nading[35] as "technical" and "apolitical." While a CHW model without the core role of advocacy would still provide care, this worker would essentially be hindered by authoritative forces and would no longer be able to challenge or seek other means to circumvent unjust workings of the broader political economic environment.

Although Medicaid reimbursement is tied to the professional citizenship of these workers and ostensibly a huge boon, it is possible that this could reduce the ability for CHWs' participation in advocacy due to the fact that current reimbursable services are strictly health focused. As such, the "non-health" associated roles fulfilled by CHWs are (and will likely be) diminished and devalued in favor of reimbursable services. If diminished in such a way, it is possible that the foundation of the CHW model will be shifted in favor of a strictly medical-focused worker. As the current verbiage of the policy states, it will "not provide reimbursement for CHW services: enrollment assistance, case management, advocacy efforts," employers are not likely to want their employees performing these activities while at work. However, the American Medical Association (AMA) and the UnitedHealth Group have developed a set of billable codes that cover issues related to the social determinants of health.[36] The AMA and UnitedHealth Group encourage the adoption of these codes that reimburse, for example, transportation for a dialysis patient.[37] Failing to value the impact of advocacy as a form of caregiving (particularly as a skill that aids clients in identifying social determinants of health and developing skills to overcome them) will hinder the full potential that CHWs could foster in improving health and well-being and potentially sacrifice a foundational aspect of this position.

Parsing out advocacy related to the level of impact is one means of rethinking the potential of this role. Although previous scholarship has assessed the varying ways in which advocacy creates impacts on society,[38] arranging advocacy as demonstrated in this book provides a different means of conceptualizing advocacy especially for policy-makers, employers, and other stakeholders. Potential employers and policy-makers who may be hesitant to include advocacy (often due to its conflation with activism) can view the various ways CHWs participate in advocacy and the direct ways it can generate salubrious outcomes on health and well-being. These stake-holders can also see how not all macro-level advocacy entails activism and, while organizing and participating in town halls and other political associ-ated events is entirely within the purview of employers to ban during work hours, allow CHWs to mobilize the community such as planning events (e.g., health fairs, community, and/or cultural festivals). This represents another way for CHWs to promote social health and connect the community. CHW participation in collaborations and coalitions improves outreach, unites com-munity members, organizes health fairs, and impacts health in macro and nonpolitical ways.

Advocacy at the professional level also yields crucial insights related to how CHWs advocate within the professional realm. This level of advocacy consists of two distinctions: (1) in which CHWs have to advocate to other professionals and stakeholders regarding their legitimacy, and (2) advocating to their own employers for their professional needs and programs provided to their communities. Advocating at this level highlights the professional needs of CHW employees as well as documenting the potential impacts of cutting a program. This type of advocacy can also highlight the self-care needs and systemic support required by these workers to be successful. Policy-makers, (potential) employers, and other stakeholders can be notified of these issues and needs through the professional-level advocacy of these workers.

Ultimately, it is vital that advocacy be reconceptualized as a form of care-giving[39] and its role within the CHW model through professionalization is protected. Stakeholders must recognize the contributions of this unique role performed by CHWs and understand its impacts at the micro, macro, and professional levels and how advocacy conducted at these levels can invoke positive outcomes for health and well-being—of individual clients, the broader community, and CHWs themselves. Additional activities should be added to the reimbursable services that include time spent with clients advocating and identifying social determinants of health and developing strategies to achieve their goals and overcome these structural forces. Taking these steps will enshrine the role of advocacy and incentivize its role for employers.

COMBATING BURNOUT AND COMPASSION FATIGUE AND PROMOTING SELF-CARE

Chapter 6 examined the effects of experiencing burnout and compassion fatigue. These deleterious conditions affect not only the ability of the CHW to do their job but also negatively impact their own health and well-being. A variety of factors contributed to the burnout and compassion fatigue experienced by these workers including job stress, lack of available resources (or difficulty in procuring them), and challenging clients. However, participants described a variety of self-care strategies that they could draw on in order to combat the effects of these conditions. Nonetheless, this was not always enough for participants and many still reported high levels of stress.

Participants were at particular risk due to the intimate and caring nature of the CHW approach. Several CHWs described not taking care of themselves in the pursuit of providing care to their clients and community. This close connection with clients also puts CHWs at risk of exposure to secondary trauma, which is especially exacerbated for those with high caseloads. Workplace stress, high caseloads, and secondary trauma contributed to burnout and compassion fatigue, compromising the ability of these workers to provide care. Self-care becomes one crucial practice among participants to diminish the effects of these deleterious conditions that can have mental and physical health implications.

Some CHWs, as a strategy of self-care, employed tough love with clients who did not seemingly become empowered. This topic was divisive, with many participants arguing that tough love is unreconcilable within CHW caregiving. Instead, tough love was only to be employed with family members and loved ones. Professional boundaries that CHWs are to maintain would thus prevent this relationship from forming between clients and CHWs and thus make the use of tough love not within the CHW repertoire of services. And, although many of the self-care strategies were idiosyncratic, employers, policy-makers, and other stakeholders must be cognizant of how they can support the self-care needs of these workers.

In helping CHWs avoid these conditions and through supporting self-care strategies, stakeholders can help diminish the deleterious effects caused by burnout and compassion fatigue. However, it is essential that policy-makers, employers, and potential employers not only support CHWs in practicing self-care but also by instituting policies that reduce burnout, recognize compassion fatigue in their workers, and provide additional resources. Employers should consider offering paid mental health days, providing a "mental health hour" (i.e., time set aside for CHWs to decompress), and establishing realistic case-loads for these workers are some actionable steps that can be implemented.

ENVISIONING THE FUTURE OF THE CHW MODEL IN INDIANA AND THE UNITED STATES

The future of the CHW model and its sustainability remains to be seen in Indiana. Several steps have put the model into motion that includes professionalization done through legislation, policy development, and Medicaid reimbursement. These steps also combined with the state-supported certification program and were all important means of removing barriers and boundaries, thereby providing this workforce with professional citizenship. Some positive news emerged following the implementation of these steps and at the conclusion of data collection. Several participants informed me that a few hospitals located in large cities in Indiana, including Fort Wayne and Indianapolis, began hiring CHWs. Other organizations were catching on to the fact that particular services were being reimbursed and the CHW title was becoming a bit more common. While there is still uncertainty—such as how professionalization will impact the CHW workforce—there are several key areas in which the CHW model can be adapted or embedded within.

One of the most versatile aspects of the CHW model is its adaptability—this model can be employed across racial and ethnic groups, gender identity, sexual orientation, individuals experiencing homelessness, substance use disorders, and/ or mental health disorders. Moreover, these workers can collaboratively work within hospitals, clinics, and social service organizations. Other first responders (e.g., firefighters, emergency medical technicians [EMTs]) can also undergo the certification training to learn the CHW approach to care. The CHW organization I collaborated with trained (and certified) a group of EMTs. There had also been talks about cross-training other first responders as well. However, those plans fell through and have yet to be discussed again. There were several important points that emerged in conducting these trainings with first responders: (1) expanding awareness of the CHW model, (2) demonstrating the unique CHW approach to care, and (3) planting a seed in these organizations to show how hiring a full-time CHW would complement the work of these first responders.

However, this also skirts a dangerous line. In cross-training first responders as CHWs, the goal must not be reductionist in approach, for example, by transforming the CHW model into a certification that can be "in addition" to another certification but rather as a means to enhance and shift the focus of each of these first responders' approach to those they help. Hiring a CHW to work with these first responders may also be beneficial through their knowledge of the community and having a different skill set compared to first responders. CHWs could go on calls with police, firefighters, and EMTs to help those in their time of need and address other needs of the family aside from the person(s) suffering the emergency.

Aside from enhancing the skill set of first responders, spreading awareness of the model, and the potential for hiring CHWs within these organizations, the need for increasing institutional and organizational support for the CHW workforce will be another potential means for job development. Given that many of the communities within which CHWs work are in need of job opportunities, the CHW model serves to not only enhance health outcomes but also as an economic opportunity. This position could possibly serve as a stepping stone for individuals to advance through the medical professional ladder, for example, transitioning from CHW to medical assistant to a registered nurse (RN) to becoming a physician associate or medical doctor (MD). However, organizations and employers must be cognizant of the cost of certification and/ or specialty trainings as these could serve as financial barriers to entering this profession. Employers and organizations must offer financial support in the form of scholarships, grants, or other options to subsidize the cost of the tuition to complete the certification course in addition to providing income for the duration of the two-week course. These steps will help ensure the CHW position is attainable and financially feasible for future CHWs.

Building on the adaptability of the model and the broad applicability of the training, the time appears ripe for the integration of these workers within the broader health and social services workforce. This book builds upon a myriad of studies that have argued for the potential of CHWs as a fully fledged member of the healthcare team and/or in patient-centered medical homes.[40] There is also large-scale, private interest in the roles that CHWs may play within the realm of health care. In May 2018, Indiana's pharmaceutical giant Eli Lilly and Company invested 7 million dollars to bring global health initiatives to address issues of diabetes through the use of CHWs in several communities within Indianapolis in a pilot study.[41] This demonstrates the interest generated via the incorporation of these workers as valued and legitimate members of the healthcare workforce. While the CHW workforce is still in its nascency in terms of its professionalization, there is significant potential that could have positive reverberations throughout the healthcare landscape of the United States.

DILEMMAS AND UNANSWERED QUESTIONS

There are a variety of dilemmas and unanswered questions provoked from the findings presented in this book. As discussed in chapter 2, there are issues that arise when a client seemingly does not want to become empowered. How to approach this situation was still a matter of debate among CHWs. Similarly, when to cut off a client or end provision of care was a difficult subject for many participants and was intimately connected to burnout and compassion fatigue. For some CHWs who were new to the profession and had just completed the certification, there were little to no opportunities to find employment as a CHW. This led to feelings of disillusionment and frustration, as evidenced by the stories of Miguel and Ximena. For other CHWs, little pay, ill-defined responsibilities, and lack of job security could produce a negative synergy when coupled with a client who refuses to take steps toward self-sufficiency. Further assessing and unpacking these negative factors may yield findings that could inform policies to better serve CHWs.

Of course, when encountering difficult clients, it could become easy for CHWs to fall into a similar trap of medical professionals when they label patients as "noncompliant," without fully understanding the structural factors that impede their health behaviors. While I have presented this dilemma from the perspective of the CHW, it is vital to understand this issue from the perspective of the client as well to fully understand the moral economy of care in which these actors operate. Asking clients such questions as "How does the CHW affect your well-being? What were your experiences prior to receiving help from a CHW? How can the CHW better serve your needs?" and more will help paint a fuller picture of the CHW-client relationship. In illuminating this side of the CHW-client relationship, additional insights can be gained to improve caregiving and better inform policy.

Other dilemmas include assessing the ramifications regarding the professionalization of this workforce in Indiana, particularly the impacts of certification and Medicaid reimbursement. Potential ramifications could include the production of a CHW hierarchy[42] that may lead to preferential hiring of certified CHWs over non-certified, serve as a barrier to entering the workforce (due to the cost of the certification course), and differential salaries determined by certification. Medicaid reimbursement for a set of CHW-specific services was an important step forward. However, this fails to reimburse for core CHW roles such as time spent with clients to identify and overcome social determinants of health and advocacy. Thus, questions arise such as (1) how will Medicaid reimbursement affect these workers? and (2) how will reimbursement potentially shift the roles of certified CHWs?

Tied closely to this will be potential future policy development regarding CHWs—will more CHWs be included in these discussions or not? How will this (or the total lack of additional policy development) impact the CHW workforce and their future in the state? As legislative steps have led to a greater integration of the CHW model, how will their inclusion within the neoliberal healthcare workforce transform their roles and approach to care-giving? These questions remained at least for the CHW workforce in Indiana. However, many of these same questions can be applied in studies assessing CHWs in other countries.

FUTURE RESEARCH DIRECTIONS

There are several areas for future research directions that studies on the topic of CHWs should consider in Indiana, the United States, and abroad. One of the most prominent means of attracting the attention of state governments, public health organizations, and potential employers is through demonstrating the cost-effectiveness and/or return-on-investment. These studies will demonstrate the cost-savings that these workers can offer within the neoliberal nature of the healthcare system, especially in the United States. A variety of studies have demonstrated the potential for short-term cost-effectiveness, cost-effectiveness in health outreach programs, and potential for long-term cost-effectiveness,[43] which serve as important complementary justifications alongside the myriad of public health studies that demonstrate the qualitative and quantitative positive health outcomes of CHWs. Additionally, future research should also include a qualitative component to further assess how various factors impact the experiences of CHWs engaged in this cost- (and life-) saving care. Future studies could attempt to quantify the impact of participation in advocacy in terms of cost-savings projections from the services of CHWs in terms of preventing illness within the workforce and cost-savings for employers since hiring CHWs.

Future research should also continue to explore the positive outcomes of CHWs on reducing the rates of, impacts of, and costs associated with issues including chronic diseases, hospital readmission rates, impact of social determinants of health, improving health equity, and other specific health outcomes. These studies should be presented to state departments of health and policy-makers to help expand awareness of and impact of these workers.

As the arguments in this book have presented, qualitative research produces valuable insights regarding CHWs and elucidates the nuances of their lived experience. Moreover, future research must include CHWs in collaborative approaches. Other scholars have asserted for the need to include these workers as research partners within data collection.[44] Fostering these collaborative relationships will help with buy-in from CHWs and their communities and improve the internal validity of findings.

Additionally, future studies should continue to assess the moral economy of care within which CHWs and their communities exist to contribute to both academic and applied research. Understanding the moral drive, obligation, motivation, and character traits that comprise the CHW workforce can help inform recruitment searches, tailor trainings for CHWs, and improve our understanding of the moral economy. Since the majority of these workers are significantly shaped by their socioeconomic status, racial/ethnic background, and other specific political economic forces, understanding how the local moral economy of care is produced and influenced is vital in policy development regarding this workforce. Other scholars have asserted how taking into account criteria such as communal congruence, trust, knowledge of resources, and ability to engender participant empowerment should be considered in measuring CHW effectiveness along with qualifications such as certification and training.[45]

Lastly, future studies should consider integrating visual methods in their approach such as photovoice. These methods produce compelling, participant-driven findings and can be used to reach the public through public forums, in marketing campaigns, and in documentaries. Visual methods can increase the reach of the findings from these projects, potentially influencing policy-makers and spreading awareness of these workers. Additionally, in pairing visual methods with collaborative approaches, CHWs serve as co-researchers, elevating their voices and allowing them to capture their lived experiences visually. These findings can elucidate the plethora of issues facing CHWs in their daily work, the impact of social determinants of health, as well as the successes that CHWs engender within their clients. These findings can then be used to influence medical professionals, policy-makers, and the broader public.

"PEOPLE NEED TO BE SEEN": A FINAL WORD

In my conversations with Lucía, I asked if there was anything she would like to say regarding the future of the CHW workforce. She emphasized the power of CHWs to serve as a witness—in other words, providing validation serves as a core contribution that CHWs offer to their clients and communities. Lucía elaborated on her vision of CHWs:

I see CHWs as an army of healers. [T]hey have the power to touch an aloneness that no one else can . . . I want there to be an army of healers . . . I witness your life and your life is worth something to me . . . to tell that to people. So I think our biggest ache in this nation is that people are not seen, there are not enough relationships—too much Facebook and social media—with all these thousands of friends and no one to see *you*. People need to be seen and that's what a CHW can do. I'm glad and very humbled and blessed that God has put me in this place for this time that we can grow that army because it's needed.

According to Lucía, CHWs serve as a positive force, a witness that sees, understands, validates, and advocates on behalf of others to demonstrate their deservingness to the world. And, through advocacy, in particular, these workers foster and elevate deservingness through connecting people to resources, care, and social, mental, and physical well-being. Leticia also offered some powerful thoughts regarding these workers, drawing on her decades of experience as a CHW:

I'd like to add that it's been a pleasure . . . to not only be a community health worker but guide, lead, and nurture community health workers because they are special. And there is something that is—like when you have something special—you've never realized that flower that was in the garden. . . . That flower in the garden that was there but you've never seen it before, you've never recognized it or realized how it makes the garden more beautiful . . . that is how I see community health workers.

Leticia's words capture the present yet invisible nature of CHWs in Indiana. In taking measures to incorporate CHWs, while enshrining their unique contributions and roles in policy, these workers may one day fulfill Lucía's and Leticia's visions. In nurturing CHWs, they have a chance to truly stand out and become the beautiful flower described by Leticia and, through their dedication and service provided to their communities, advocate for justice, address the social determinants of health, and strive for the health equity that their communities—and all people—deserve.

NOTES

1. See, e.g., Brodwin 2008, 2010, 2011; Buch 2013, 2014; Davis-Floyd and Davis 1996; Maes 2017; Maupin 2011, 2015; Zigon 2011.
2. U.S. Bureau of Labor Statistics 2018, see https://www.bls.gov/oes/2018/may/oes211094.htm. Other studies have estimated the CHW population of the U.S. to be between 85,000 to 200,000 (Perry et al. 2014).

3. Ibid.

4. See e.g., Romero and Bhatt 2021 and Snavely 2016.

5. See https://www.who.int/health-topics/health-workforce#tab=tab_1.

6. See https://www.ruralhealthweb.org/getattachment/Advocate/Policy -Documents/HealthCareWorkforceDistributionandShortageJanuary2012.pdf.aspx ?lang=en-US.

7. Logan and Castañeda 2020.

8. U.S. Bureau of Labor Statistics 2020.

9. Ibid.

10. See Shamasunder et al. 2020

11. Lopez, Hart, and Katz 2020.

12. CDC 2021.

13. Ballard et al. 2020, CDC 2020, Goldfield et al. 2020, Peretz et al. 2020.

14. Johnson et al. 2013, Maes et al. 2014, Nebeker et al. 2020.

15. Bourgois 1998, Fassin 2005, Horton 2015, Maes 2017, Nading 2013, Swartz 2013.

16. Bourgois 1998.

17. Bourgois and Schonberg 2009.

18. Horton 2015.

19. Zabiliūtė 2021: 29.

20. Swartz and Colvin 2015.

21. Nading 2013.

22. Adams 1998; Butler, Chillas, and Muhr 2012; Dahle 2012; Witz 1992.

23. Berthold 2016, Brownstein et al. 2011, George et al. 2020, Ingram et al. 2020, Rosenthal et al. 2010, Rush 2012.

24. Rosenthal et al. 2010.

25. Ibid.

26. Balcazar et al. 2011, Catalani et al. 2009, Ingram et al. 2014.

27. Rosenthal et al. 2010: 1340.

28. See, e.g., Colvin and Swartz 2015; Closser 2015; Maes 2015, 2017; Nading 2013.

29. See https://apha.org/policies-and-advocacy/public-health-policy-statements/ policy-database/2015/01/28/14/15/support-for-community-health-worker-leadership.

30. C3 Project 2018.

31. Catalani et al. 2009, Closser et al. 2019, Ingram et al. 2020, Pérez and Martinez 2008, Rosenthal et al. 2011, Sabo et al. 2013, Sugarman et al. 2021, Wennerstrom et al. 2021.

32. Nading 2013, Pérez and Martinez 2008.

33. See the Introduction for a brief explanation of liberation theology, also Pérez and Martinez 2008.

34. Cupertino et al. 2013; Pérez and Martinez 2008; Wiggins et al. 2009, 2013, 2014.

35. Nading 2013.

36. Japsen 2019.

37. For more information, see https://newsroom.uhc.com/content/uhc/newsroom/news-releases/AMA-announcement.html.

38. Sabo et al. 2013.

39. Logan and Castañeda 2020.

40. See, e.g., Balcazar et al. 2011, Chin et al. 2012, Findley et al. 2014, Kangovi et al. 2015, Reinschmidt et al. 2015, Shah et al. 2014.

41. Fisher 2018b, Rudavsky 2018, Russell 2018.

42. Maupin 2011.

43. See, e.g., Allen et al. 2014, Brown et al. 2012, Cross-Barnet et al. 2018, Fedder et al. 2003, Gaziano et al. 2014, Vaughan et al. 2015.

44. Maes et al. 2014, Nebeker et al. 2020, Pérez and Martinez 2008.

45. Islam et al. 2017.

References

Adams, Ann, Realpe, Alba, Vail, Laura, Buckingham, Christopher D., Erby, Lori H., and Debra Roter. "How Doctors' Communication Style and Race Concordance Influence African-Caribbean Patients when Disclosing Depression." *Patient Education & Counseling* 98, no. 10 (2015): 1266–1273.

Adams, Richard E., Boscarino, Joseph A., and Charles R. Figley. "Compassion Fatigue and Psychological Distress Among Social Workers: A Validation Study." *American Journal of Orthopsychiatry* 76, no. 1 (2006): 103–108.

Adams, Tracey L. "Combining Gender, Class, and Race: Structuring Relations in the Ontario Dental Profession." *Gender & Society* 12, no. 5 (1998): 578–597.

Alkema, Karen, Linton, Jeremy M., and Randall Davies. "A Study for the Relationship Between Self-Care, Compassion Satisfaction, Compassion Fatigue, and Burnout Among Hospice Professionals." *Journal of Social Work in End-of-Life & Palliative Care* 4, no. 2 (2008): 101–119.

Allen, Jerilyn K., Dennison Himmelfarb, Cheryl R., Szanton, Sarah L., and Kevin D. Frick. "Cost-effectiveness of Nurse Practitioner/Community Health Worker Care to Reduce Cardiovascular Health Disparities." *Journal of Cardiovascular Nursing* 29, no. 4 (2014): 308–314.

America's Health Rankings. "Indiana–Annual Report." 2020. Accessed June 21, 2020. https://www.americashealthrankings.org/explore/annual/state/IN.

American Immigration Council. "New Americans in Indiana: The Political and Economic Power of Immigrants, Latinos, and Asians in the Hoosier State." 2015. Accessed Sep. 15, 2020. https://www.americanimmigrationcouncil.org/research/immigrants-in-indiana.

———. "Immigrants in Indiana." 2017. Accessed Sep. 15, 2020. https://www.americanimmigrationcouncil.org/sites/default/files/research/immigrants_in_indiana.pdf.

American Public Health Association (APHA). "Support for Community Health Worker Leadership in Determining Workforce Standards for Training and Credentialing." 2014. Accessed Sep. 15, 2020. https://www.apha.org/policies-and

-advocacy/public-health-policy-statements/policy-database/2015/01/28/14/15/support-for-community-health-worker-leadership.

———. "Community Health Workers." 2021. Accessed Apr. 28, 2021. https://www.apha.org/apha-communities/member-sections/community-health-workers

Artiga, Samantha, and Elizabeth Hinton. "Beyond Health Care: The Role of Social Determinants in Promoting Health and Health Equity." 2018. Accessed June 23, 2021. https://www.kff.org/disparities-policy/issue-brief/beyond-health-care-the-role-of-social-determinants-in-promoting-health-and-health-equity/.

Arvey, Sarah R., Fernandez, Maria E., LaRue, Denise M., and L. Kay Bartholomew. "When *Promotoras* and Technology Meet: A Qualitative Analysis of *Promotoras'* Use of Small Media to Increase Cancer Screening Among South Texas Latinos." *Health Education & Behavior* 39, no. 3 (2012): 352–363.

Backe, Emma L. "A Crisis of Care: The Politics and Therapeutics of a Rape Crisis Hotline." *Medical Anthropology Quarterly* 32, no. 4 (2018): 463–480.

Bade, Bonnie, and Konane Martinez. "Full Circle: The Method of Collaborative Anthropology for Regional and Transnational Research." In *Migration and Health: A Research Methods Handbook*. Edited by Schenker, Marc B., Castañeda, Xóchitl, and Alfonso Rodriguez-Lainz, 306–326. Berkeley: University of California Press, 2014.

Balcazar, Hector, Rosenthal, E. Lee, Brownstein, J. Nell, Rush, Carl H., Matos, Sergio, and Lorenza Hernandez. "Community Health Workers Can Be a Public Health Force for Change in the United States: Three Actions for a New Paradigm." *American Journal of Public Health* 101, no. 12 (2011): 2199–2203.

Ballard, Madeleine, Bancroft, Emily, Nesbit, Josh, Johnson, Ari, Holeman, Isaac, Foth, Jennifer … and Daniel Palazuelos. "Prioritising the Role of Community Health Workers in the COVID-19 Response." *BMJ Global Health* 5, no. 6 (2020): e002550.

Baquero, Barbara, Goldman, Shira N., Simán, Florence, Muqueeth, Sadiya, Eng, Eugenia, and Scott D. Rhodes. (2014). "'Mi Cuerpo, Nuestro Responsabilidad': Using Photovoice to Describe the Assets and Barriers to Sexual and Reproductive Health among Latinos." *Journal of Health Disparities & Research Practice* 7, no. 1 (2014): 65–83.

Berthold, Tim, ed. *Foundations for Community Health Workers*. San Francisco: Jossey-Bass, 2016.

Besterman-Dahan, Karen, Lind, Jason D., and Theresa Crocker. "'You Never Heard Jesus Say To Make Sure You Take Time Out For Yourself': Military Chaplains and the Stigma of Mental Illness." *Annals of Anthropological Practice* 37, no. 2 (2014): 108–129.

Bhutani, Jaikrit, Bhutani, Sukriti, Singh Balhara, Yatan Pal, and Sanjay Kalra. "Compassion Fatigue and Burnout Amongst Clinicians: A Medical Exploratory Study." *Indian Journal of Psychological Medicine* 34, no. 4 (2012): 332–337.

Bijari, Bita, and Ali Abassi. "Prevalence of Burnout Syndrome and Associated Factors Among Rural Health Workers (Behvarzes) in South Khorasan." *Iranian Red Crescent Medical Journal* 18, no. 10 (2016): e25390.

Blanchard, Janice, Nayar, Shakti, and Nicole Lurie. "Patient-Provider and Patient-Staff Racial Concordance and Perceptions of Mistreatment in the Health Care Setting." *Journal of General Internal Medicine* 22, no. 8 (2007): 1184–1189.

Bourgois, Philippe. "The Moral Economies of Homeless Heroin Addicts: Confronting Ethnography, HIV Risk, and Everyday Violence in San Francisco Shooting Encampments." *Substance Use & Misuse* 33, no. 11 (1998): 2323–2351.

Bourgois, Philippe, and Jeffrey Schonberg. *Righteous Dopefiend*. Berkeley: University of California Press, 2009.

Bovbjerg, Randall B., Eyster, Lauren, Ormond, Barbara A., Anderson, Theresa, and Elizabeth Richardson. "Opportunities for Community Health Workers in the Era of Health Reform." 2013. Accessed Sep. 15, 2020. http://www.urban.org/sites/default/files/alfresco/publication-pdfs/413071-Opportunities-for-Community-Health-Workers-in-the-Era-of-Health-Reform.PDF.

Brodwin, Paul. "The Coproduction of Moral Discourse in U.S. Community Psychiatry." *Medical Anthropology Quarterly* 22, no. 2 (2008): 127–147.

———. "The Assemblage of Compliance in Psychiatric Case Management." *Anthropology & Medicine* 17, no. 2 (2010): 129–143.

———. "Futility in the Practice of Community Psychiatry." *Medical Anthropology Quarterly* 25, no. 2 (2011): 189–208.

Brown III, H. Shelton, Wilson, Kimberly J.; Pagán, José A., Arcari, Christine M., Martinez, Martha, Smith, Kirk, and Belinda Reininger. "Cost-Effectiveness Analysis of a Community Health Worker Intervention for Low-Income Hispanic Adults with Diabetes." *CDC Preventing Chronic Disease* 9 (2012): 1–9.

Brownstein, J. Nell, Bone, Lee R., Dennison, Cheryl R., Hill, Martha N., Kim, Myong T., and David M. Levine. "Community Health Workers as Interventionists in the Prevention and Control of Heart Disease and Stroke." *American Journal of Preventive Medicine* 29, no. 5 S1 (2005): 128–133.

Buch, Elana. D. "Senses of Care: Embodying Inequality and Sustaining Personhood in the Home Care of Older Adults in Chicago." *American Ethnologist* 40, no. 4 (2013): 637–650.

———. "Troubling Gifts of Care: Vulnerable Persons and Threatening Exchanges in Chicago's Home Care Industry." *Medical Anthropology Quarterly* 28, no. 4 (2014): 599–615.

Butler, Nick, Chillas, Shiona, and Sara Louise Muhr. "Professions at the Margins." *Ephemera* 12, no. 3 (2012): 259–272.

Catalani, Caricia E. C., Findley, Sally E., Matos, Sergio, and Romelia Rodriguez. "Community Health Worker Insights on their Training and Certification." *Progress in Community Health Partnerships: Research, Education, and Action* 3, no. 3 (2009): 227–235.

Centers for Disease Control and Prevention (CDC). "Resources for Community Health Workers, Community Health Representatives, and Promotores de la Salud." 2020. Accessed June 16, 2021. https://www.cdc.gov/coronavirus/2019-ncov/hcp/community-health-workers/index.html.

———. "Health Equity Considerations and Racial and Ethnic Minority Groups." 2021. Accessed June 17, 2021. https://www.cdc.gov/coronavirus/2019-ncov/community/health-equity/race-ethnicity.html.

Charlot, Marjory, Santana, M. Christina, Chen, Clara A., Bak, Sharon, Heeren, Timothy C., Battaglia, Tracy A., Egan, Patrick A., Kalish, Richard, and Karen

M. Freund. "Impact of Patient and Navigator Race and Language Concordance on Care After Cancer Screening Abnormalities." *Cancer* 121, no. 9 (2015): 1477–1483.

Chávez, Jorge M., Engelbrecht, Christine M., Lopez, Anayeli, Viramontez Anguiano, Ruben P., and J. Roberto Reyes. "Collateral Consequences: The Impact of Local Immigration Policies on Latino Immigrant Families in North Central Indiana." In *Outside Justice: Immigration and the Criminalizing Impact of Changing Policy and Practice.* Edited by Brotherton, David C., Stageman, Daniel L., and Shirley P. Leyro. New York: Springer, 2013.

Cherrington, Andrea, Ayala, Guadalupe X., Elder, John P., Arredondo, Elva M., Fouad, Mona, and Isabel Scarinci. "Recognizing the Diverse Roles of Community Health Workers in the Elimination of Health Disparities: From Paid Staff to Volunteers." *Ethnicity & Disease* 20, no. 2 (2010): 189–194.

Chin, Marshall H., Clarke, Amanda R., Nocon, Robert S., Casey, Alicia A., Goddu, Anna P., Keesecker, Niciole M., and Scott C. Cook. "A Roadmap and Best Practices for Organizations to Reduce Racial and Ethnic Disparities in Health Care." *Journal of General Internal Medicine* 27, no. 8 (2012): 992–1000.

Choi, Elizabeth. "Getting to Know Our Neighbors, the Burmese Community on the South Side." 2016. Accessed June 23, 2021. https://www.wishtv.com/news/getting -to-know-our-neighbors-the-burmese-community-on-the-south-side/.

CHW Central. "Women in the Changing World of Community Health Work." 2017. Accessed February 21, 2021. https://chwcentral.org/twg_article/women-in-the -changing-world-of-community-health-work/.

Closser, Svea. "Pakistan's Lady Health Worker Labor Movement and the Moral Economy of Heroism." *Annals of Anthropological Practice* 39, no. 1 (2015): 16–28.

Closser, Svea, and Rashid Jooma. "Why We Must Provide Better Support for Pakistan's Female Frontline Health Workers." *PLOS Medicine* 10, no. 10 (2013): e100128.

Closser, Svea, Napier, Harriet, Maes, Kenneth, Abesha, Roza, Gebremariam, Hana, Backe, Grace, Fossett, Sarah, and Yihenew Tesfaye. "Does Volunteer Community Health Work Empower Women? Evidence from the Women's Development Army." *Health Policy & Planning* 34, no. 4 (2019): 298–306.

Coaston, Susannah C. "Self-Care Through Self-Compassion: A Balm for Burnout." *The Professional Counselor* 7, no. 3 (2017): 285–297.

Colvin, Christopher J., and Swartz, Alison. "Extension Agents or Agents of Change? Community Health Workers and the Politics of Care Work in Postapartheid South Africa." *Annals of Anthropological Practice* 39, no. 1 (2015): 29–41.

Community Health Worker Core Consensus Project (C3). "Together Leaning Toward the Sky." 2018. Accessed Sep. 15, 2020. https://0d6c00fe-eae1-492b-8e7d-80acec-b5a3c8.filesusr.com/ugd/7ec423_2b0893bcc93a422396c744be8c1d54d1.pdf.

Contreras, Ricardo, Larson, Kim, Pierpont, John, Griffith, David, and Juvencio Rocha-Peralta. "Capacity Building in the Latino Community: Lessons from the Promotora Project in Eastern North Carolina." *Practicing Anthropology* 34, no. 4 (2012): 19–23.

Corbin, Juliet, and Anselm Strauss. *Basics of Qualitative Research* (3rd Edition). Thousand Oaks: Sage, 2008.

Cross-Barnet, Caitlin, Ruiz, Sarah, Skillman, Morgan, Dhopeshwarkar, Rina, Friedman Singer, Rachel, Carpenter, Rachel, Freij, Maysoun, Campanella, Suzanne, Page Snyder, Lynne, and Erin Colligan. "Higher Quality at Lower Cost: Community Health Worker Interventions in the Health Care Innovation Awards." *Journal of Health Disparities Research and Practice* 11, no. 2 (2018). 150–164.

Cupertino, A. Paula, Suarez, Natalia, Sanderson Cox, Lisa, Fernández, Cielo, Jaramillo, Mary Lou, Morgan, Aura, Garrett, Susan, Mendoza, Irazema, and Edward F. Ellerbeck. "Empowering Promotores de Salud to Engage in Community-Based Participatory Research." *Journal of Immigrant & Refugee Studies* 11, no. 1 (2013): 24–43.

Dahle, Rannveig. "Social Work: A History of Gender and Class in the Profession." *Ephemera* 12, no. 3 (2012): 309–326.

Davenport, Beverly A. "Witnessing and the Medical Gaze: How Medical Students Learn to See at a Free Clinic for the Homeless." *Medical Anthropology Quarterly* 14, no. 3 (2000): 310–327.

Davis-Floyd, Robbie, and Elizabeth Davis. "Intuition as Authoritative Knowledge in Midwifery and Homebirth." *Medical Anthropology Quarterly* 10, no. 2 (1996): 237–269.

De Hert, Stefan. "Burnout in Healthcare Workers: Prevalence, Impact and Preventative Strategies." *Local & Regional Anesthesia* 13 (2020): 171–183.

Deitrick, Lynn M., Paxton, Hannah D., Rivera, Alicia, Gertner, Eric J., Biery, Nyann, Letcher, Abby S., Lahoz, Lissette M., Maldonado, Edgardo, and Debbie Salas-Lopez. "Understanding the Role of the Promotora in a Latino Diabetes Education Program." *Qualitative Health Research*, 20, no. 3 (2010): 386–399.

Enard, Kimberly R., and Deborah M. Ganelin. "Reducing Preventable Emergency Department Utilization and Costs by Using Community Health Workers as Patient Navigators." *Journal of Healthcare Management* 58, no. 6 (2013): 412–428.

Encalada, Lorena, Quizphe, Arturo, Andrade, Diana, and María Merchán. "El Rol de Los Promotores En El Uso y Abuso de Los Antibioticos." *Ateneo* 20, no. 1 (2019): 29–44.

Fassin, Didier. "Compassion and Repression: The Moral Economy of Immigration Policies in France." *Cultural Anthropology* 20, no. 3 (2005): 362–387.

———. *Humanitarian Reason: A Moral History of the Present.* Translated by Rachel Gomme. Berkeley: University of California Press, 2012.

———. "Children as Victims: The Moral Economy of Childhood in the Times of AIDS." In *When People Come First.* Edited by Biehl, João, and Adriana Petryna. Princeton: Princeton University Press, 2013.

Fedder, Donald O., Chang, Ruyu J., Curry, Sheila, and Gloria Nichols. "The Effectiveness of a Community Health Worker Outreach Program on Healthcare Utilization of West Baltimore City Medicaid Patients with Diabetes, With or Without Hypertension." *Ethnicity & Disease* 13, no. 1 (2003): 22–27.

Findley, Sally, Matos, Sergio, Hicks, April, Chang, Ji, and Douglas Reich. "Community Health Worker Integration Into the Health Care Team Accomplishes the Triple Aim in a Patient-Centered Medical Home: A Bronx Tale. *Journal of Ambulatory Care Management* 37, no. 1 (2014): 82–91.

Fisher, Kristin. "How Death Doulas Can Help People at the End of Their Life." 2018a. Accessed on Sept. 15, 2020. from https://www.healthline.com/health-news /how-death-doulas-can-help-people-at-the-end-of-their-life#1.

Fisher, Nicole. "Eli Lilly Takes $7M Gamble on Global Health Working…In Indiana." 2018b. Accessed on June 24, 2021. https://www.forbes.com/sites/nicole-fisher/2018/05/14/eli-lilly-takes-7m-gamble-on-global-health-working-in-indiana/ ?sh=797db0865748

Foucault, Michel. *The Birth of the Clinic: An Archaeology of Medical Perception.* New York: Vintage Books, 1994 [1973].

Galtung, Johan. *Peace: Research, Education, Action.* Copenhagen: Christian Eljers, 1975.

Garfield, Rachel, Orgera, Kendal, and Anthony Damico. "The Uninsured and the ACA: A Primer – Key Facts about Health Insurance and the Uninsured Amidst Changes to the Affordable Care Act." 2019. Accessed on March 20, 2020. https:// www.kff.org/report-section/the-uninsured-and-the-aca-a-primer-key-facts-about -health-insurance-and-the-uninsured-amidst-changes-to-the-affordable-care-act -how-many-people-are-uninsured/.

Gaziano, Thomas A., Bertram, Melanie, Tollman, Stephen M., and Karen J. Hofman. 2014. "Hypertension Education and Adherence in South Africa: A Cost-Effectiveness Analysis of Community Health Workers." *BMC Public Health*, 14 no. 240 (2014): 1–9.

Ge, Cuixia, Fu, Jialiang, Chang, Ying, and Lie Wang. "Factors Associated with Job Satisfaction among Chinese Community Health Workers: A Cross-Sectional Study." *BMC Public Health* 11, no. 884 (2011): 1–13.

George, Rani, Gunn, Rose, Wiggins, Noelle, Rowland, Ruth, Davis, Melinda M., Maes, Kenneth, Kuzma, Angie, and K. John McConnell. "Early Lessons and Strategies from Statewide Efforts to Integrate Community Health Workers in Medicaid." *Journal of Health Care for the Poor & Underserved* 31, no. 2 (2020): 845–858.

Getrich, Christina, Heying, Shirley, Willging, Cathleen, and Howard Waitzkin. "An Ethnography of Clinic 'Noise' in a Community-based, Promotora-centered Mental Health Intervention." *Social Science & Medicine* 65 (2007): 319–330.

Goldade, Kathryn. "'Health Is Hard Here' or 'Health for All?' The Politics of Blame, Gender, and Health Care for Undocumented Nicaraguan Migrants in Costa Rica." *Medical Anthropology Quarterly* 23, no. 4 (2009): 483–503.

Goldfield, Norbert I., Crittenden, Robert, Fox, Durrell, McDonough, John, Nichols, Len, and E. Lee Rosenthal. "COVID-19 Crisis Creates Opportunities for Community-Centered Population Health: Community Health Workers at the Center." *Journal of Ambulatory Care Management* 43, no. 3 (2020): 184–190.

Gómez, Sofía, and Heide Castañeda. "'Recognize Our Humanity': Immigrant Youth Voices on Health Care in Arizona's Restrictive Political Environment." *Qualitative Health Research* 29, no. 4 (2018): 498–509.

Good, Byron J., Fischer, Michael M. J., Willen, Sarah S., and Mary-Jo DelVecchio Good, eds. *A Reader in Medical Anthropology: Theoretical Trajectories, Emergent Realities.* Malden: Wiley-Blackwell Publishing, 2010.

Goodnough, Abby. "What Has Mike Pence Done in Health?" 2020. Accessed February 27, 2020. https://www.nytimes.com/2020/02/27/health/pence-coronavirus-indiana.html.

Groppe, Maureen. "Uninsured Rate Continues to Drop Indiana Under Obamacare." 2017. Accessed Sept. 15, 2020. https://www.indystar.com/story/news/politics/2017/09/13/uninsured-rate-continues-drop-indiana-under-obamacare/659146001/.

Haq, Zaeem, Iqbal, Zafar, and Atif Rahman. "Job Stress Among Community Health Workers: A Multi-Method Study from Pakistan." *International Journal of Mental Health Systems* 2, no. 1 (2008): 15–20.

Holmes, Seth, and Heide Castañeda. "Ethnographic Research in Migration and Health." In *Migration and Health: A Research Methods Handbook.* Edited by Schenker, Marc B., Castañeda, Xóchitl, and Alfonso Rodriguez-Lainz, 265–277. Berkeley: University of California Press, 2014.

Horn, David J., and Catherine B. Johnston. "Burnout and Self-Care for Palliative Care Practitioners." *Medical Clinics of North America* 104, no. 3 (2020): 561–572.

Horton, Sarah. "Identity Loan: The Moral Economy of Migrant Document Exchange in California's Central Valley." *American Ethnologist* 42, no. 1 (2015): 55–67.

Indiana State Department of Health. "Community Health Workers (CHWs)." 2016. Accessed Sep. 15, 2020. https://www.in.gov/isdh/24942.htm.

Ingram, Maia, Sabo, Samantha, Redondo, Floribella, Soto, Yanitza, Russell, Kim, Carter, Heather, Bender, Brooke, and Jill Guernsey De Zapien. "Establishing Voluntary Certification of Community Health Workers in Arizona: A Policy Case Study of Building a Unified Workforce." *Human Resources for Health* 18, no. 1 (2020): 46.

Ingram, Maia, Sabo, Samantha, Rothers, Janet, Wennerstrom, Ashley, and Jill Guernsey de Zapien. "Community Health Workers and Community Advocacy: Addressing Health Disparities." *Journal of Community Health* 33, no. 6 (2008): 417–424.

Ingram, Maia, Schachter, Ken A., Sabo, Samantha J., Reinschmidt, Kerstin. M., Gomez, Sofia, Guernsey De Zapien, Jill, and Scott C. Carvajal. "A Community Health Worker Intervention to Address the Social Determinants of Health Through Policy Change." *Journal of Primary Prevention* 35 (2014): 119–123.

Islam, Nadia, Shapiro, Ephraim, Wyatt, Laura, Riley, Lindsey, Zanowiak, Jennifer, Ursua, Rhodora, and Chau Trinh-Shevrin. "Evaluating Community Health Workers' Attributes, Roles, and Pathways of Action in Immigrant Communities." *Preventive Medicine* 103 (2017): 1–7.

Japsen, Bruce. "AMA Backs UnitedHealth's Billing Codes for Social Determinants of Health." 2019. Accessed Sept. 15, 2020. https://www.forbes.com/sites/brucejapsen/2019/04/02/ama-backs-unitedhealths-billing-codes-for-social-determinants-of-health/#4f54b1fc2204

Johnson, Cassandra, Sharkey, Joseph R., Dean, Wesley R., St. John, Julie A., and Maria Castillo. "*Promotoras* as Research Partners to Engage Health Disparity

Communities." *Journal of the Academy of Nutrition & Dietetics* 113, no. 5 (2013): 638–642.

Kane, Erin P., Collinsworth, Ashley W., Schmidt, Kathryn L., Brown, Rachel M., Snead, Christine A., Barnes, Sunni A., Fleming, Neil S. and James W. Walton. "Improving Diabetes Care and Outcomes with Community Health Workers." *Family Practice* 33, no. 5 (2016): 523–528.

Kangovi, Shreya, Grande, David, and Chau Trinh-Shevrin. "From Rhetoric to Reality—Community Health Workers in Post-Reform U.S. Health Care." *New England Journal of Medicine* 372, no. 24 (2015): 2277–2279.

Katigbak, Carina, Van Devanter, Nancy, Islam, Nadia., and Chau Trinh-Shevrin. "Partners in Health: A Conceptual Framework for the Role of Community Health Workers in Facilitating Patient's Adoption of Healthy Behaviors." *American Journal of Public Health* 105, no. 5 (2015): 872–880.

Katzen, Amy, and Maggie Morgan. "Affordable Care Act Opportunities for Community Health Workers: How Medicaid Preventive Services, Medicaid Health Homes, and State Innovation Models are Including Community Health Workers." Center for Health Law and Policy Innovation at Harvard Law School. 2014. Accessed Sept. 15, 2020. http://www.chlpi.org/wp-content/uploads/2013/12/ACA -Opportunities-for-CHWsFINAL-8-12.pdf.

Kleinpell, Ruth, Moss, Marc, Good, Vicki, Gozal David, and Curtis Sessler. "The Critical Nature of Addressing Burnout Prevention: Results from the Critical Care Societies Collaborative's National Summit and Survey on Prevention and Management of Burnout in the ICU." *Critical Care Medicine* 48, no. 2 (2020): 249–253.

Krieger, James W., Takaro, Tim K., Song, Lin, and Marcia Weaver. "The Seattle-King County Healthy Homes Project: A Randomized, Controlled Trial of a Community Health Worker Intervention to Decrease Exposure to Indoor Asthma Triggers." *American Journal of Public Health* 95, no. 4 (2015): 652–659.

Kumar, Disha, Schlundt, David G., and Kenneth A. Wallston. "Patient-Physician Race Concordance and Its Relationship to Perceived Health Outcomes." *Ethnicity & Disease* 19, no. 3 (2009): 345–351.

Langhout, Regina Day. "Photovoice as Methodology." In *Migration and Health: A Research Methods Handbook*. Edited by Schenker, Marc B., Castañeda, Xóchitl, and Alfonso Rodriguez-Lainz, 327–342. Berkeley: University of California Press, 2014.

Lawson, Gerard, and Jennifer M. Cook. "Wellness, Self-care, and Burnout Prevention." In *Clinical Mental Health Counseling: Elements of Effective Practice*. Edited by J. Scott Young & Craig S. Cashwell, 313–335. New York: Sage Publications, Inc., 2017.

Lehmann, Uta, and David Sanders. "Community Health Workers: What Do We Know About Them?" 2007. Accessed Sept. 15, 2020. http://www.who.int/hrh/ documents/community_health_workers.pdf

Li, Li, Hu, Hongyan, Zhou, Hao, He, Changzhi, Fan, Lihua, Liu, Xinyan, Zhang, Zhong, Li, Heng, and Tao Sun. "Work Stress, Work Motivation and Their Effects on Job Satisfaction in Community Health Workers: A Cross-Sectional Survey in China." *BMJ Open* 4, no. 6 (2014): e004897.

Ligenza, Linda. "Compassion Fatigue and Self-Care." 2018. Accessed April 22, 2020. https://integration.samhsa.gov/pbhci-learning-community/Compassion _Fatigue_Office_Hours.pdf.

Livingston, Julie. *Improvising Medicine: An African Oncology Ward in an Emerging Cancer Epidemic*. Durham: Duke University Press, 2012.

Lo, Ming-Cheng M., and Emerald T. Nguyen. "Resisting the Racialization of Medical Deservingness: How Latinx Nurses Produce Symbolic Resources for Latinx Immigrants in Clinical Encounters." *Social Science & Medicine* 270 (2021): 113677.

Logan, Ryan I. "Not a Duty But an Opportunity: Exploring the Lived Experiences of Community Health Workers in Indiana through Photovoice." *Qualitative Research in Medicine & Healthcare* 2, no. 3 (2018): 132–144.

———. "Being A Community Health Worker Means Advocating: Participation, Perceptions, and Challenges in Advocacy." *Anthropology in Action* 26, no. 2 (2019): 9–18.

———. "'A Poverty in Understanding': Assessing the Structural Challenges Experienced by Community Health Workers and Their Clients." *Global Public Health* 15, no. 1 (2020): 137–150.

———. "Professionalization as a 'Double-Edged Sword': Assessing the Professional Citizenship of Community Health Workers in the Midwest." *Human Organization* 80, no. 3 (2021): 192–202.

Logan, Ryan I. and Heide Castañeda. "Addressing Health Disparities in the Rural United States: Advocacy as Caregiving among Community Health Workers and *Promotores de Salud*." *International Journal of Environmental Research & Public Health* 17: 9223.

Lopez, Leo, Hart, Louis H., and Mitchell H. Katz. "Racial and Ethnic Health Disparities Related to COVID-19." *Journal of the American Medical Association* 325, no. 8 (2021): 719–720.

Maes, Kenneth. "Volunteerism or Labor Exploitation? Harnessing the Volunteer Spirit to Sustain AIDS Treatment Program." *Human Organization* 71, no. 1 (2012): 54–64.

———. "Community Health Workers and Social Change: An Introduction." *Annals of Anthropological Practice* 39, no. 1 (2015a): 1–15.

———. "'Volunteers Are Not Paid Because They Are Priceless': Community Health Worker Capacities and Values in an AIDS Treatment Intervention in Urban Ethiopia." *Medical Anthropology Quarterly* 29, no. 1 (2015b): 97–115.

———. "Experts' Tools, Altruists, and Job-Seekers: Visions of Community Health Workers in Ethiopia's Antiretroviral Centre of Excellence." *Critical African Studies* 8, no. 3 (2016): 335–349.

———. *The Lives of Community Health Workers: Local Labor and Global Health in Urban Ethiopia*. New York: Routledge, 2017.

Maes, Kenneth, and Ippolytos Kalofonos. "Becoming and Remaining Community Health Workers: Perspectives from Ethiopia and Mozambique." *Social Science & Medicine* 87 (2013): 52–59.

Maes, Kenneth, and Selamawit Shifferaw. "Cycles of Poverty, Food Insecurity, and Psychosocial Stress Among AIDS Care Volunteers in Urban Ethiopia." *Annals of Anthropological Practice* 35, no. 1 (2011): 98–115.

Maes, Kenneth, Closser, Svea, and Ippolytos Kalofanos. "Listening to Community Health Workers: How Ethnographic Research Can Inform Positive Relationships Among Community Health Workers, Health Institutions, and Communities." *American Journal of Public Health* 104, no. 5 (2014): e5–e9.

Maes, Kenneth, Closser, Svea, Vorel, Ethan, and Yihenew Tesfaye. "Using Community Health Workers: Discipline and Hierarchy in Ethiopia's Women's Development Army." *Annals of Anthropological Practice* 39, no. 1 (2015a): 42–57.

———. "A Women's Development Army: Narratives of Community Health Worker Investment and Empowerment in Rural Ethiopia." *Studies in Comparative International Development* 50, no. 4 (2015b): 455–478.

Malakouti, Seyed Kazem, Nojomi, Marzieh, Salehi, Maryam, and Bita Bijari. "Job Stress and Burnout Syndrome in a Sample of Rural Health Workers, Behvarzes, in Tehran, Iran." *Iranian Journal of Psychiatry* 6, no. 2 (2011): 70–74.

Manson, Aaron. "Language Concordance as a Determinant of Patient Compliance and Emergency Room Use in Patients with Asthma." *Medical Care* 26, no. 12 (1988): 1119–1128.

Maricopa County Department of Public Health. "Community Health Workers Opportunities and the Affordable Care Act (ACA)." 2013. Accessed June 23, 2021. http://coveraz.org/wp-content/uploads/2013/09/Community-Health-Workers.pdf.

Marrow, Helen, B. "Deserving to a Point: Unauthorized Immigrants in San Francisco's Universal Access Healthcare Model." *Social Science & Medicine* 74, no. 6 (2012): 846–854.

Maslach, Christina, and Michael P. Leiter. "New Insights into Burnout and Health Care: Strategies for Improving Civility and Alleviating Burnout." *Medical Teacher* 39, no. 2 (2017): 160–163.

Maupin, Jonathan N. "Divergent Models of Community Health Workers in Highland Guatemala." *Human Organization* 70, no. 1 (2011): 44–53.

———. "Shifting Identities: The Transformation of Community Health Workers in Highland Guatemala." *Annals of Anthropological Practice* 39, no. 1 (2015): 73–88.

Mayfield-Johnson, Susan, Rachal, John R., Butler III, James. "'When We Learn Better, We Do Better': Describing Changes in Empowerment through PhotoVoice among Community Health Advisors in a Breast and Cervical Cancer Health Promotion Program in Mississippi and Alabama." *Adult Education Quarterly* 64, no. 2 (2014): 91–109.

Mays, Glen P. and Sharla A. Smith. Evidence Links Increases in Public Health Spending to Declines in Preventable Deaths. *Health Affairs* 30, no. 8 (2011): 1585–1593.

Meghani, Salimah H., Brooks, Jacqueline M., Gipson-Jones, Trina, Waite, Roberta, Whitfield-Harris, Lisa, and Janet A. Deatrick. "Patient-Provider Race-Concordance: Does It Matter in Improving Minority Patients' Health Outcomes?" *Ethnicity & Health* 14, no. 1 (2009): 107–130.

Mitchell, Claudia, DeLange, Naydene, Moletsane, Relebohile, Stuart, Jean, and Thabisile Buthelezi. "Giving a Face to HIV and AIDS: On the Uses of Photo-voice by Teachers and Community Health Care Workers Working with Youth in Rural South Africa." *Qualitative Research in Psychology* 2, no. 3 (2005): 257–270.

Mirambeau, Alberta M., Wang, Guijing, Ruggles, Laural, and Diane O. Dunet. "A Cost Analysis of a Community Health Worker Program in Rural Vermont." *Journal of Community Health* 38, no. 6 (2013): 1050–1057.

Mota, Caroline M., Dosea, Giselle S., and Paula S. Nunes. "Avaliação da presença da Síndrome de *Burnout* em Agentes Comunitários de Saúde no município de Aracaju, Sergipe, Brasil." *Ciência & Saúde Coletiva* 19, no. 12 (2014): 4719–4726.

Motta, Robert W. "Secondary Trauma." *International Journal of Emergency Mental Health* 10, no. 4 (2008): 291–298.

Murayama, Hiroshi, Spencer, Michael S., Sinco, Brandy R., Palmisano, Gloria, and Edith C. Kieffer. "Does Racial/Ethnic Identity Influence the Effectiveness of a Community Health Worker Intervention for African American and Latino Adults with Type 2 Diabetes?" *Health Education & Behavior* 44, no. 3 (2017): 485–493.

Musoke, David, Ssemugabo, Charles, Ndejjo, Rawlance, Molyneux, Sassy, and Elizabeth Ekirapa-Kiracho. "Ethical Practice In My Work: Community Health Workers' Perspectives using Photovoice in Wakiso District, Uganda." *BMC Medical Ethics* 21, no. 1 (2020): 68.

Nading, Alex. "'Love Isn't There in Your Stomach': A Moral Economy of Medical Citizenship among Nicaraguan Community Health Workers." *Medical Anthropology Quarterly* 27, no. 1 (2013): 84–102.

———. *Mosquito Trails: Ecology, Health, and the Politics of Entanglement.* Berkeley: University of California Press, 2014.

Nebeker, Camille, Giacinto, Rebeca Espinoza, Pacheco, Blanca Azucena, López-Arenas, Araceli and Michael Kalichman. "Prioritizing Competences for 'Research' Promotores and Community Health Workers." *Health Promotion Practice* 22, no. 4 (2020): 512–523.

Nebeker, Camille, Kalichman, Michael, Talavera, Ana, and John Elder. "Training in Research Ethics and Standards for Community Health Workers and Promotores Engaged in Latino Health Research." *Hastings Center Report* 45, no. 4 (2015): 20–27.

Nichter, Mark. *Global Health: Why Cultural Perceptions, Social Representations, and Biopolitics Matter.* Tucson: University of Arizona Press, 2008.

O'Donovan, James, Hamala, Rebecca, Namanda, Allan S., Musoke, David, Ssemugabo, Charles, and Niall Winters. "'We Are the People Whose Opinions Don't Matter': A Photovoice Study Exploring Challenges Faced by Community Health Workers in Uganda." *Global Public Health* 15, no 3 (2020): 384–401.

Peretz, Patricia J., Islam, Nadia, and Luz Adriana Matiz. "Community Health Workers and COVID-19—Addressing Social Determinants of Health in Times of Crisis and Beyond." *New England Journal of Medicine* 383, no. 19 (2020): e108.

Pérez, Leda M., and Jacqueline Martinez. "Community Health Workers: Social Justice and Policy Advocates for Community Health and Well-Being." *American Journal of Public Health* 98, no. 1 (2008): 11–14.

Pérez-Escamilla, Rafael, Garcia, Jonathan, and David Song, D. "Health Care Access Among Hispanic Immigrants: *¿Alguien Está Escuchando?* [Is Anybody Listening?]." *NAPA Bulletin* 34, no. 1 (2010): 47–67.

Perry, Henry B., Zulliger, Rose, and Michael M. Rogers. "Community Health Workers in Low-, Middle-, and High-Income Countries: An Overview of Their History, Recent Evaluation, and Current Effectiveness." *Annual Review of Public Health* 35 (2014): 399–421.

Pew Research Center. "U.S. Unauthorized Immigrant Population Estimates by State, 2016." Accessed Sept. 15, 2020. http://www.pewhispanic.org/interactives/unauthorized-immigrants/.

Powell, Tara, and Paula Yuma-Guerrero. "Supporting Community Health Workers After a Disaster: Findings from a Mixed-Methods Pilot Evaluation Study of Psychoeducational Intervention." *Disaster Medicine & Public Health Preparedness* 10, no. 5 (2016): 754–761.

Price, Sara. "Professionalizing Midwifery: Exploring Medically Imagined Labor Rooms in Rural Rajasthan." *Medical Anthropology Quarterly* 28, no. 4 (2014): 519–536.

Prince, Ruth. "HIV and the Moral Economy of Survival in an East African City." *Medical Anthropology Quarterly* 26, no. 4 (2012): 534–556.

Puente, Michael. "Burmese Refugees Find New Home in Indiana." 2007. Accessed June 23, 2021. https://www.npr.org/templates/story/story.php?storyId=14841071.

Quesada, James, Hart, Laurie K., and Philippe Bourgois. "Structural Vulnerability and Health: Latino Migrant Laborers in the United States." *Medical Anthropology* 30, no. 4 (2011): 339–362.

Ramirez-Valles, Jesus. "Promoting Health, Promoting Women: The Construction of Female and Professional Identities in the Discourse of Community Health Workers." *Social Science & Medicine* 47, no. 11 (1998): 1749–1762.

Reinschmidt, Kerstin M., Ingram, Maia, Schachter, Kenneth, Sabo, Samantha, Verdugo, Lorena, and Scott Carvajal. "The Impact of Integrating Community Advocacy Into Community Health Worker Roles on Health-Focused Organization and Community Health Workers in Southern Arizona." *Journal of Ambulatory Care Management* 38, no. 3 (2015): 244–253.

Robert Wood Johnson Foundation. "New County Health Rankings Show Differences in Health and Opportunity by Place and Race." 2018. Accessed June 23, 2021. https://www.rwjf.org/en/library/articles-and-news/2018/03/county-health-rankings-show-differences-in-health-by-place-and-race.html.

Romero, Laura and Jay Bhatt. "Pandemic Has Made Shortage of Health Care Workers Even Worse, Say Experts." 2021. Accessed June 16, 2021. https://abcnews.go.com/US/pandemic-made-shortage-health-care-workers-worse-experts/story?id=77811713.

Rosenthal, E. Lee, Brownstein J. Nell, Rush, Carl H., Hirsch Gail R., Willaert, Anne M., Scott, Jacqueline R., Holderby, Lisa R., and Durrell J. Fox. "Community Health Workers: Part of the Solution." *Health Affairs* 29, no. 7 (2010): 1338–1342.

Rosenthal, E. Lee, Wiggins, Noelle, Ingram, Maia, Mayfield-Johnson, Susan, and Jill Guernsey De Zapien. "Community Health Workers Then and Now: An Overview of National Studies Aimed at Defining the Field." *Journal of Ambulatory Care* 34, no. 3 (2011): 247–259.

Rudavsky, Shari. "Lilly Gives $7M to 'Where You Live Shouldn't Determine How Long You Live' Pilot Program." 2018. Accessed Sept. 16, 2020 https://www.indy-star.com/story/news/2018/05/01/lilly-iupui-partner-7-m-project-address-diabetes-low-income-areas/566696002/.

Rudowitz, Robin, Musumeci, MaryBeth, and Elizabeth Hinton. "Digging Into the Data: What Can We Learn from the State Evaluation of Healthy Indiana (HIP 2.0) Premiums." 2018. Accessed Sept. 16, 2020. https://www.kff.org/medicaid/issue-brief/digging-into-the-data-what-can-we-learn-from-the-state-evaluation-of-healthy-indiana-hip-2-0-premiums/.

Rush, Carl H. "Return on Investment from Employment of Community Health Workers." *Journal of Ambulatory Care* 35, no. 2 (2012): 133–137.

Russ, Ann Julienne. "Love's Labor Paid for: Gift and Commodity at the Threshold of Death." *Cultural Anthropology* 20, no 1 (2005): 128–155.

Russell, John. "Major Health Initiative Targets 3 Indianapolis Neighborhoods with High Diabetes Rates." 2018. Accessed Sept. 16, 2020. https://www.ibj.com/articles/68628-major-health-initiative-targets-3-indianapolis-neighborhoods-with-high-diabetes-rates.

Ryabov, Igor. "Cost-effectiveness of Community Health Workers in Controlling Diabetes Epidemic on the U.S.-Mexico Border." *Public Health* 128, no. 7 (2014): 636–642.

Sabo, Samantha, Flores, Melissa, Wennerstrom, Ashley, Bell, Melanie L., Verdugo, Lorena, Carvajal, Scott, and Maia Ingram. "Community Health Workers Promote Civic Engagement and Organizational Capacity to Impact Policy." *Journal of Community Health* 42, no. 6 (2017): 1197–1203.

Sabo, Samantha, Ingram, Maia, Reinschmidt, Kerstin M., Schachter, Kenneth, Jacobs, Laurel, Guernsey de Zapien, Jill., Robinson, Laurie, and Scott Carvajal. "Predictors and a Framework for Fostering Community Advocacy as a Community Health Worker Core Function to Eliminate Health Disparities." *American Journal of Public Health* 103, no. 7 (2013): e67–e73.

Sabo, Samantha, Wennerstrom, Ashley, Phillips, David, Haywoord, Catherine, Redondo, Floribella, Bell, Melanie L., and Maia Ingram. "Community Health Worker Professional Advocacy." *Journal of Ambulatory Care Management* 38, no. 3 (2015): 225–235.

Salloum, Alison, Kondrat, David C., Johnco, Carly, and Kayla R. Olson. "The Role of Self-Care on Compassion Satisfaction, Burnout and Secondary Trauma among Child Welfare Workers." *Children & Youth Services Review* 49 (2015): 54–61.

Sanders, Michelle, Winters, Paul, and Kevin Fiscella. "Preliminary Validation of a Scale to Measure Patient Perceived Similarity to their Navigator." *BMC Research Notes* 8 (2015): 388.

Sansó, Noemí, Galiana, Laura, Oliver, Amparo, Pascual, Antonio, Sinclair, Shane, and Enric Benito. "Palliative Care Professionals' Inner Life: Exploring the Relationships Among Awareness, Self-Care, and Compassion Satisfaction with Fatigue, Burnout, and Coping with Death." *Journal of Pain & Symptom Management* 50, no. 2 (2015): 200–207.

Schmit, Cason D., Washburn, David J., LaFleur, Megan, Martinez, Denise, Thompson, Emily, and Timothy Callaghan. "Community Health Worker Sustainability: Funding, Payment, and Reimbursement Laws in the United States." *Public Health Reports* (2021): Online ahead of print.

Schoenthaler, Antoinette, Allegrante, John P., Chaplin, William, and Gbenga Ogedegbe. "The Effect of Patient-Provider Communication on Medication Adherence in Hypertensive Black Patients: Does Race Concordance Matter?" *Annals of Behavioral Medicine* 43, no. 3 (2012): 372–382.

Scott, James. *The Moral Economy of the Peasant: Rebellion and Subsistence in Southeast Asia.* New Haven: Yale University Press, 1976.

Selamu, Medhin, Thornicroft, Graham, Fekadu, Abebaw, and Charlotte Hanlon. "Conceptualisation of Job-Related Wellbeing, Stress and Burnout among Healthcare Workers in Rural Ethiopia: A Qualitative Study." *BMC Health Services Research* 17, no. 1 (2017): 412–422.

Semuels, Alana. "Indiana's Medicaid Experiment May Reveal Obamacare's Future." 2016. Accessed Sep. 16, 2020. https://www.theatlantic.com/business/archive/2016/12/medicaid-and-mike-pence/511262/.

Shah, Megha, Heisler, Michele, and Matthew Davis. "Community Health Workers and the Patient Protection and Affordable Care Act: An Opportunity for Research, Advocacy, and Policy Agenda." *Journal of Health Care for the Poor and Underserved* 25, no. 1 (2014): 17–24.

Shamasunder, Sriram, Holmes, Seth M., Goronga, Tinashe, Carrasco, Hector, Katz, Elyse, Frankfurter, Raphael, and Salmaan Keshavjee. "COVID-19 Reveals Weak Health Systems by Design: Why We Must Re-Make Global Health in this Historic Moment." *Global Public Health* 15, no. 7: 1083–1089.

Shepherd-Banigan, Megan, Hohl, Sarah D., Vaughan, Catalina, Ibarra, Genoveva, Carosso, Elizabeth, and Beti Thompson. "The Promotora Explained Everything": Participant Experiences During a Household-Level Diabetes Education Program." *The Diabetes Educator* 40, no. 4 (2014): 507–515.

Sherwen, Laurie N., Schwolsky-Fitch, Elena, Rodriguez, Romelia, Horta, Greg and Ivanna Lopez. "The Community Health Worker Cultural Mentoring Project: Preparing Professional Students for Team Work with Health Workers from Urban Communities." *Journal of Allied Health* 36, no. 1 (2007): e66-e86.

Snavely, Timothy M. "A Brief Economic Analysis of the Looming Nursing Shortage in the United States." *Nursing Economic$* 34, no. 2 (2016): 98–100.

Stevenson, Lisa. *Life Beside Itself: Imagining Care in the Canadian Arctic.* Berkeley: University of California Press, 2014.

Sugarman, Meredith, Ezouah, Pascaline, Haywoord, Catherine, and Ashley Wennerstrom. "Promoting Community Health Worker Leadership in Policy Development: Results from a Louisiana Workforce Study." *Journal of Community Health* 46, no. 1 (2021): 64–74.

Swartz, Alison. "Legacy, Legitimacy, and Possibility: An Exploration of Community Health Worker Experience across the Generations in Khayelitsha, South Africa." *Medical Anthropology Quarterly* 27, no. 2 (2013): 139–154.

Swartz, Alison and Christopher J. Colvin. "'It's In Our Veins': Caring Natures and Material Motivations of Community Health Workers in Contexts of Economic Marginalisation." *Critical Public Health* 25, no. 2 (2015): 139–152.

Takasugi, Tomo and Andrew Lee. "Why Do Community Health Workers Volunteer?" A Qualitative Study in Kenya." *Public Health* 126, no. 10 (2012): 839–845.

Tantchou, Josiane. "Poor Working Conditions, HIV/AIDS and Burnout: A Study in Cameroon." *Anthropology in Action* 21, no. 3 (2014): 31–42.

Taylor, Marla, Nowaskie, Dustin Z., and Alan Witchey. LGBTQ+ Community Needs: 2020 Indianapolis. 2020. Accessed May 24, 2021. https://www.document-cloud.org/documents/6956121-LGBTQ-Community-Survey-Report.html?embed=true&responsive=false&sidebar=false.

Thompson, E. P. "The Moral Economy of the English Crowd in the Eighteenth Century." *Past & Present* 50 (1971): 76–136.

Traylor, Ana H., Schmittdiel, Julie A., Uratsu, Connie S., Mangione, Carol M. Mangione, and Usha Subramanian. "Adherence to Cardiovascular Disease Medications: Does Patient-Provider Race/Ethnicity and Language Concordance Matter?" *Journal of General Internal Medicine* 25, no. 11 (2010): 1172–1177.

Tripathy, Jaya P., Goel, Sanu, and Ajay M. V. Kumar. "Measuring and Understanding Motivation among Community Health Workers in Rural Health Facilities in India: A Mixed Method Study." *BMC Health Services Research* 16 (2016): 366.

Turgoose, David and Lucy Maddox. "Predictors of Compassion Fatigue in Mental Health Professionals: A Narrative Review." *Traumatology* 23, no. 2 (2017): 172–185.

U.S. Bureau of Labor Statistics. "Occupational Employment and Wages, May 2017 – 21-1094 Community Health Workers." 2018. Accessed Sep. 15, 2020. https://www.bls.gov/oes/current/oes211094.htm.

———. "Health Educators and Community Health Workers." 2020. Accessed April 3, 2020. https://www.bls.gov/ooh/community-and-social-service/health-educators.htm.

U.S. Census Bureau. "QuickFacts – Indiana." 2019a. Accessed May 13, 2021. https://www.census.gov/quickfacts/in.

———. "QuickFacts – Indiana; Indianapolis City (Balance), Indiana." 2019b. Accessed May 13, 2021. https://www.census.gov/quickfacts/fact/table/IN,indianapoliscitybalanceindiana/PST045219.

U.S. Department of Health and Human Services (HHS). "Community Health Worker National Workforce Survey" 2007. Accessed May 12, 2021. https://bhw.hrsa.gov/sites/default/files/bureau-health-workforce/data-research/community-health-work-force.pdf.

Valen, Mieca, Narayan, Suzanne, and Lorene Wedeking. "An Innovative Approach to Diabetes Education for a Hispanic Population Utilizing Community Health Workers." *Journal of Cultural Diversity* 19, no. 1 (2012): 10–17.

van de Ruit, Catherine. "Unintended Consequences of Community Health Worker Programs in South Africa." *Qualitative Health Research* 29, no. 11 (2019): 1535–1548.

Vaughan, Kelsey, Kok, Maryse C., Witter, Sophie, and Marjolein Dieleman. "Costs and Cost-Effectiveness of Community Health Workers: Evidence from a Literature Review." *Human Resources for Health* 13 (2015): 71.

Viladrich, Anahí. "Beyond Welfare Reform: Reframing Undocumented Immigrants' Entitlement to Health Care in the United States, A Critical Review." *Social Science & Medicine* 74, no. 6 (2012): 822–829.

Villa-Torres, Laura, Fleming, Paul J., and Clare Barrington. "Engaging Men as Promotores de Salud: Perceptions of Community Health Workers Among Latino Men in North Carolina." *Journal of Community Health* 40, no. 1 (2015): 167–174.

Viswanathan, Meera, Kraschnewski, Jennifer L., Nishikawa, Brett, Morgan, Laura C., Honeycutt, Amanda A., Thieda, Patricia, Lohr, Kathleen N., and Daniel E. Jonas. "Outcomes and Costs of Community Health Worker Interventions: A Systematic Review." *Medical Care* 48, no. 9 (2010): 792–808.

Wailoo, Keith, Livingston, Julie, and Peter J. Guarnaccia. *A Death Retold: Jessica Santillan, the Bungled Transplant, and Paradoxes of Medical Citizenship.* Chapel Hill: The University of North Carolina Press, 2006.

Walton, James W., Snead, Christine A., Collinsworth, Ashley W., and Kathryn L. Schmidt. "Reducing Diabetes Disparities Through the Implementation of a Community Health Worker-Led Diabetes Self-Management Education Program." *Family & Community Health* 35, no. 2 (2012): 161–171.

Wang, Caroline. "Photovoice: A Participatory Action Research Strategy Applied to Women's Health." *Journal of Women's Health* 8, no. 2 (1999): 185–192.

Wang, Caroline, and Mary Ann Burris. "Photovoice: Concept, Methodology, and Use for Participatory Needs Assessment." *Health Education & Behavior* 24, no. 3 (1997): 369–387.

Wasserman, Joan, Palmer, Richard C., Gomez, Marcia M., Berzon, Rick, Ibrahim, Said A., and John Z. Ayanian. "Advancing Health Services Research to Eliminate Health Care Disparities." *American Journal of Public Health* 109, no. S1 (2019): S64–S69.

Watters, Charles. "Refugees at Europe's Borders: The Moral Economy of Care." *Transcultural Psychiatry* 44, no. 3 (2007): 394–417.

Wells, Kristen J., Luque, John S., Miladinovic, Branko, Vargas, Natalia, Asvat, Yasmin, Roetzheim, Richard G., and Ambuj Kumar. "Do Community Health Worker Interventions Improve Rates of Screening Mammography in the United States? A Systematic Review." *Cancer, Epidemiology, Biomarkers & Prevention* 20, no. 8 (2011): 1580–1598.

Wennerstrom, Ashley, Sugarman, Meredith, Rush, Carl, Barbero, Collee, Jayapul-Philip, Bina, Fulmer, Erika B., Shantharam, Sharada, Moeti, Refilwe, and Theresa Mason. "'Nothing About Us Without Us': Insights from State-level Efforts to Implement Community Health Worker Certification." *Journal of Health Care for the Poor & Underserved* 32, no. 2 (2021): 892–899.

Wiggins, Noelle, Johnson, Denise, Avila, María, Farquhar, Stephanie A., Michael, Yvonne L., Rios, Teresa, and Alicia Lopez. 2009. "Using Popular Education for Community Empowerment: Perspectives of Community Health Workers in the

Poder Es Salud/Power for Health Program." *Critical Public Health* 19, no. 1 (2009): 11–22.

Wiggins, Noelle, Hughes, Adele, Rodriguez, Adriana, Potter, Catherine, and Teresa Rios-Campos. *"La Palabra Es Salud* (The Word is Health): Combining Mixed Methods and CBPR to Understand the Comparative Effectiveness of Popular Conventional Education." *Journal of Mixed Methods Research* 8, no. 3 (2014): 278–298.

Wiggins, Noelle, Kaan, Samantha, Rios-Campos, Teresa, Gaonkar, Rujuta, Morgan, Elizabeth R., and Jamaica Robinson. "Preparing Community Health Workers for Their Role as Agents of Social Change: Experience of the Community Capacitation Center." *Journal of Community Practice* 21, no. 3 (2013): 186–202.

Wilkinson, Iain and Arthur Kleinman. *A Passion for Society: How We Think About Human Suffering.* Berkeley: University of California Press, 2016.

Witz, Anne. *Professions and Patriarchy.* London, United Kingdom: Routledge, 1992.

World Health Organization (WHO). "Burn-out an 'Occupational Phenomenon': International Classification of Diseases." 2019. Accessed April 22, 2020. https://www.who.int/mental_health/evidence/burn-out/en/.

———. "What Do We Mean By Self-Care?" 2020. Accessed April 22, 2020. https://www.who.int/reproductivehealth/self-care-interventions/definitions/en/.

Zabiliūtė, Emilija. "Ethics of Neighborly Intimacy among Community Health Activists in Delhi." *Medical Anthropology* 40, no. 1 (2021): 20–34.

Zigon, Jason. 2011. "A Moral and Ethical Assemblage in Russian Orthodox Drug Rehabilitation." *Ethos* 39, no. 1 (2011): 30–50.

Index

advocacy, 2, 5, 8–10, 17–18, 35–36, 44, 52, 77, 81, 90, 95, 103, 115, 117–19, 139, 144, 155, 164–65, 171, 179, 181; as caregiving, 4, 18, 55, 136–39, 173–75; challenges in, 133–36; difficulties with clients in, 135; and engendering empowerment, 122, 125, 128, 135; fusing levels of, 128–29; impact on the medical gaze, 167; levels of, 120–21; at the macro level, 126–28, 134–36, 138, 167, 173–75; at the micro level, 121–26, 129, 134–36, 138, 173, 175; professional citizenship and, 131–32, 136, 138–39; at the professional level, 80, 128–33, 135–38, 155, 168, 173–75
American Medical Association (AMA), 174
Arizona, 6, 90, 169

barefoot doctors, 5
burnout, 10, 18, 51, 108, 133, 135, 139, 142, 160–61n5, 178; CHW experiences with, 144–48, 157; definition and description of, 143; difference from compassion fatigue, 161; impact of self-care on, 151–55; impacts of the structural violence on, 147; impacts on the well-being of CHWs by, 131, 135, 141, 147; mind-body medicine and, 159; preventing, 103, 148–51, 175–76

Calumet (River) Region, 1
case manager(s), 9, 76, 79
certification, x, 15, 17, 22n72, 28, 33, 65, 72, 79, 83, 100, 109, 131, 169, 171, 180; CHW opinions of, 88; connection to legitimizing mechanisms, 12, 73, 170; connection to professional citizenship, 84; cost of, 8, 88; description of the certification, 3, 86; description of the certification course, 1, 8–9; first responders and, 176–77; grandfathering, 88, 94n14; impacts of, 75, 86–92, 105, 132; impacts resulting from a lack of, 86; opinions of, 170; ramifications of, 77, 88–89, 97, 170, 177–78; relation to scope of care and, 95, 103, 114; skills related to self-care provided by, 141, 144, 151
Chicago, x
Children's Health Insurance Program (CHIP), 102, 136, 169
client-centered care, 157–58
community health worker(s), ix, 77, 87, 93, 130–32, 149, 181; adaptability of, 176–77; certified (CCHW), 75, 78, 84, 86, 88, 106, 171; cost-effectiveness of,

109–11, 130, 169, 179; creation
of a hierarchy of, 77, 170, 178;
critique of the term, 77; cycle
of the CHW-client relationship,
52; definition of, 1, 5; essential
qualities of, 49–50; governor's task
force on, 9, 11, 72, 93, 132, 168;
impact of certification on, 170–71;
impact of religiosity on, 32, 62–65,
152; issues of funding concerning,
7, 28, 39, 82, 96–98, 108–9, 111,
114, 129, 135, 149, 169, 172–73;
lack/loss of, 42, 137; as medical
interpreters, 81–82, 87, 95–96;
problems associated with the
multiple titles of, 7, 74–78, 81–83,
92, 131, 170; resources and, 36–41,
43; unpaid labor of, 51, 127, 145,
168; as volunteers, 83–84
Community Health Worker (CHW)
Section of the American Public
Health Association, 1, 93, 170
Community Health Workers'
Organization of Indiana (CHWOI),
3, 7–9, 15–16, 22n75, 72, 86, 88, 92,
94n14, 95, 145, 159–61; history of,
7; virtual support groups for CHWs
provided by, 161
compassion fatigue, 18, 131, 139, 156,
160–61, 175–76, 178; definition
and description of, 143; difference
from burnout, 161; impacts of the
structural violence on, 147; impacts
on the well-being of CHWs by,
147; preventing, 148–51; protective
factors against, 148
concordance, racial and ethnic, 58–60;
in the ancillary medical team, 60;
studies analyzing, 59–60
COVID-19 pandemic, 3, 8, 164

Deferred Action for Childhood Arrivals
(DACA) Program, 127–28
Department of Workforce Development,
9

deserving/ness, 4, 25, 35, 43, 68, 73, 84,
102, 136–37, 181; undeserving, 11,
55, 73, 136, 171
diabetes educators, 17
doula, 9, 12, 17, 66, 73, 80, 96, 155

East Chicago, 1
Economic Opportunity Act of 1964, 6
educação popular, 173
Eli Lilly and Company, 177
engendering empowerment, 48, 144,
146, 154, 156, 165, 180; advocacy
at the micro level and, 119, 121–22,
125, 135; building self-sufficiency
via, 48, 52–54; challenges of,
66–68, 166–68, 178; challenges with
advocacy and, 135; as a component
of advocacy, 122; critique of, 55,
68, 167; definition of, 52; impact of
gender in, 61–63; impact of shared
racial/ethnic background in, 55–60
Ethiopia, 111, 114
Evansville, 109

Federal Migrant Health Act of 1962, 6
Fort Wayne, 12, 109, 176

Gary, 1, 128
Great Society programs, 6

Hammond, 1
Health Insurance Portability and
Accountability Act (HIPAA) of
1996, 21n67, 28, 61, 99–100,
114, 172; as a boundary in CHW
caregiving, 99–100
Healthy Indiana Plan, 101
Healthy Indiana Plan 2.0 (HIP 2.0),
20n31, 99, 114–15n4, 127; critiques
of, 101
Holcomb, Eric, 9; governor, 9, 72,
168
home healthcare worker, 9
Hurricane Maria, 128
Hurricane Sandy, 159

Illinois, 1
Immigration and Customs Enforcement (ICE), 14, 122
Indianapolis, ix, 12, 24, 33, 64, 83–84, 109, 119, 122, 176–77
Indian Health Service, 6
Indiana State Department of Health (ISDH), 7, 9, 75–76, 86

Johnson, Lyndon B., 6

lactation consultant, 12
legitimizing mechanisms, 11–12, 73–75, 86, 89–91, 132, 149, 170–71; description of, 12; increasing awareness of CHWs as a, 171. *See also* professional citizenship
lesbian, gay, bisexual, transgender, queer (LGBTQ), 13–14, 63, 65, 149
liberation theology, 5–6, 173

Massachusetts, 169
Meals on Wheels, 132
Medicaid, 27–28, 42, 87, 89, 101–2, 115n4, 115nn11, 127, 136, 169; Medicaid expansion, 7, 27, 97, 99, 101, 115; Office of Medicaid Policy and Planning, 9, 90. *See also* Healthy Indiana Plan 2.0
Medicaid reimbursement, 6–7, 12, 72–73, 77, 90–92, 168–69, 173–74, 178–79; connection to the certification, 86; critiques of, 77, 90; effects on CHWs, 77, 91, 179; as a goal of the CHW task force, 168; as a legitimizing mechanism, 17, 74–75, 84, 86, 90–91, 170–71, 173, 176; in Minnesota, 169; reimbursable services, 9, 12, 28, 72–73, 75, 90, 138
medical anthropology, xi, 163
medical citizenship, 11, 35, 44, 64, 72–73, 84, 86, 102, 171
medical gaze, 34–36, 44–45n20, 55, 167
Medicare, 2, 19n7, 102

Michigan, 1
midwifery/midwives, 12, 17, 73, 74, 96
mind-body medicine, 159–60; description of, 159
Minnesota, 6, 90, 169
moral economy, 16, 35, 67, 69, 138, 180; in anthropological studies, 24, 48, 50; between CHWs and clients, 17, 138, 165, 167; definition of, 24; explanation of, 10; informing policy, 166; remuneration and the, 111
moral economy of care, 10, 16, 18, 28–30, 48–50, 53–54, 97, 115, 118, 125, 144–45, 148, 151, 155, 160–61, 163, 178; challenges and repercussions in the, 41, 43, 48, 67; definition of, 25; future studies on, 180; impact of gender on the, 61, 63; laws, policies, and structural factors shaping the, 26–29, 42, 96, 137–38, 164–65; the medical gaze and the, 36; moral division in the, 63–66; referrals and the, 51–52; remaining part of the, 32–33, 35, 44, 51, 68–69; resources and the, 36–39

Nicaragua, 35, 112

On My Way to Pre-K, 101
Oregon, 6, 90, 169

Pakistan, 114
Patient Protection and Affordable Care Act (ACA) of 2010, 7, 27–28, 75–77, 83, 90, 101, 114–15n11, 127–28, 136, 169; ACA navigator(s), 97, 124; description of, 97–99; impacts on CHWs and clients, 97–99; legitimacy provided to CHWs by, 77
Paulo Freire, 173
Pence, Mike, 14
photovoice, xi, 15–16, 21n65, 22n73, 33, 37, 54, 84–85, 100, 124, 180
Priority Enforcement Program, 14

professional citizenship, 18, 72–75, 79–84, 88–93, 96, 111, 132, 135–36, 138, 146, 151, 153, 170–73, 176; benefits of, 12; connection to legitimizing mechanisms, 74–75, 149; definition of, 11, 72; description of, 73; facilitation of, 17; impact of certification on, 86, 88, 92; impact of Medicaid reimbursement on, 84, 89–92; impact of multiple titles for CHWs and, 75, 78–79; impact of the ACA on, 98; lack of recognition and, 73, 79–81, 92; medical interpreters and, 81–82, 131; policy and, 77. *See also* legitimizing mechanisms

promotor(a)(es) [de salud], 2, 5, 42, 76, 81, 95–96, 106–7, 148

Puerto Rico, 23, 128

The Region, 1–2

scope of care/practice, 4, 8, 28, 64, 81, 95–97, 118, 129, 144, 171–72; definition of, 103; description of, 17, 95–96; establishing boundaries via, 103–8, 148, 157, 167; going outside the, 29, 93, 96, 104–8, 114, 171

secondary trauma, 142, 144, 175

Secure Communities, 13–14

self-care, 8, 18, 30, 130–31, 133, 139, 141–45, 148–54, 158–61, 174–76; benefits of, 159; challenges in practicing, 155–56; connection between caregiving and, 144, 153–55; definition of, 151; description of, 144; flexibility as a form of, 30; as a protective factor, 144; religion as, 32, 152; scope of practice as, 103; strategies of, 141–42, 148, 151–55; supporting, 158–60; tough love as a strategy of, 156–58

social determinant(s) of health, 8, 11–12, 31–34, 43–44, 77, 84, 89–90, 102, 115, 117, 121, 132, 147,

164–65, 181; advocacy to address, 136–37; CHW impacts on, 12, 31, 34, 53, 55, 82, 89, 96, 105, 123, 125; description of, 5; examples of, 11; future research on, 179–80; impacts in the moral economy of care, 43; impacts on communities served by CHWs, 26, 117, 121; Medicaid reimbursable services and, 90, 174–75, 179; transportation as a, 42–43, 105; witnessing and the, 36

structural violence, 1, 4, 14, 17, 147; addressing via advocacy, 119, 136; description of, 19n1; effects on CHWs, 11, 30, 32, 144; impact in communities served by CHWs, 26–27, 68, 73, 107, 163, 171; shared between CHWs and clients, 56

structural vulnerability, 25–27, 55–56, 58, 107, 117, 155, 160, 167; impact on care workers, 27; impact on CHWs, 11–12, 26; impact on communities serviced by CHWs, 11–12, 25, 29, 55, 114, 136–37; the medical gaze and, 36; shared, 27, 56, 84, 86, 92, 137–38, 153; in the workplace, 73, 108, 112

Supplemental Nutrition Assistance Program (SNAP), 102, 136

tough love, 18, 175–76; accountability instead of, 158, 161; description of, 156; as a form of self-care, 156–58. *See also* self-care

Trump administration, 14, 136

UnitedHealth Group, 174

white coat hypertension, 69n10

white coat syndrome, 56, 69n10. *See also* white coat hypertension

witnessing, 35–36, 44, 180–81

World Health Organization (WHO), 151, 159

About the Author

Ryan I. Logan, PhD, MPH, is an assistant professor of anthropology at California State University, Stanislaus. His research interests include medical paraprofessionals, community health workers, health disparities, migration, and complementary and alternative medicine.

www.ingramcontent.com/pod-product-compliance
Lightning Source LLC
Chambersburg PA
CBHW050646280326
41932CB00015B/2801